EXERCISE

physical activity for heart and health

by

Barbara Johnston Fletcher, RN, MN, FAHA, FPCNA, FAAN
John D. Cantwell, MD, MACP, FACC
Gerald F. Fletcher, MD, FAHA, FACC

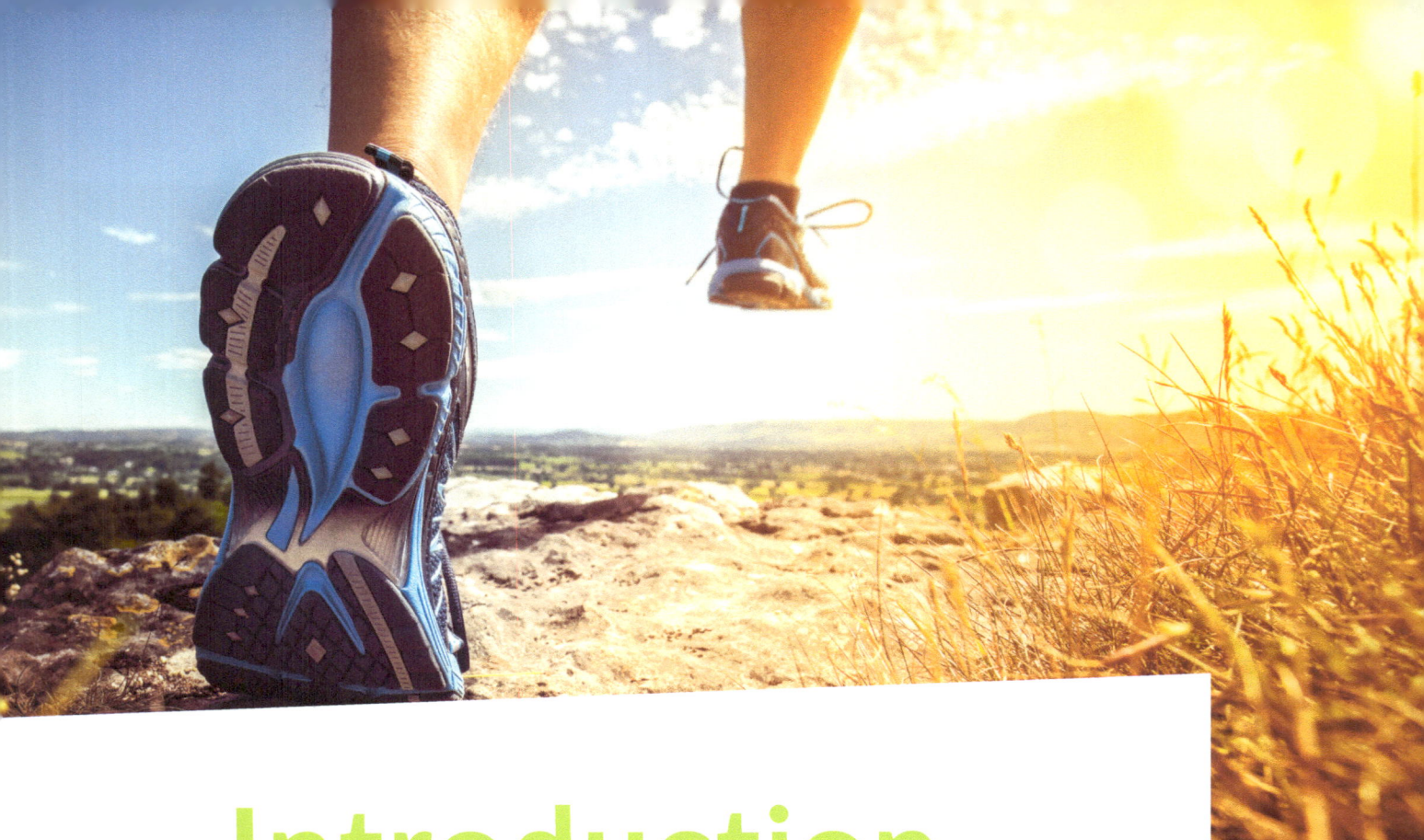

Introduction

Exercise **IS** important to your heart and health. It should be something you enjoy and can do most days for 30-60 minutes.

This book will help you make wise decisions about exercise. It will help you understand the good effects that exercise can have on your body. It also gives you actual exercise programs to try. People who already exercise can use this book as well as people who are just thinking about exercise. It can be used by people who have just had a heart attack, heart surgery, angioplasty, a stent or other heart or health problems, and by healthy people of all ages.

Before starting any regular exercises, know the exact state of your health. If you are already under a doctor's care, get his or her advice before doing any exercise. Most of all, we want you to exercise safely and have fun doing it.

Throughout this book, we will use the term "Health Care Provider" or HCP to refer to everyone involved in your care. This includes doctors, nurses, exercise physiologists, physical therapists and others.

Table of contents

continued

EXERCISE FOR HEART & HEALTH should not replace what your own health care provider (HCP) tells you about exercise. This book is to help you understand more about exercise and your heart and health.

Why exercise

It's a good way to feel good and be strong. With strong muscles and bones, you can do everyday activities easier. It also helps you look and feel good. Exercise makes you have a lower risk of heart and blood vessel disease. Regular exercise can help:

- the heart pump blood and oxygen to the body with less effort

- lower blood pressure

- lose body fat and body weight

- blood fats get better—HDL (good cholesterol) increases and triglycerides (bad fat) decrease

- other good blood changes (lower blood sugar, less harmful clotting)

- control metabolic syndrome (p.12)

- reduce mental stress, depression and anxiety

- strengthen the immune system

- reduce the risk of certain cancers (such as colon and breast)

- reduce falls in the elderly

- bone density, muscle mass, strength and balance improve

- improve blood flow to all muscles

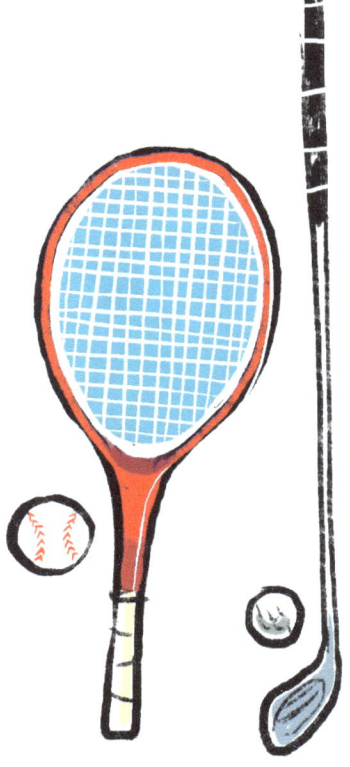

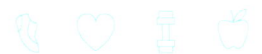

the heart and muscles

Regular exercise helps **your heart pump easier.** When you are fit, your heart can beat fewer times per minute and still get the same amount of blood and oxygen to your body. This means your heart is more efficient. As your muscles get stronger they are more able to accept and use this oxygen. In time, you notice that it takes less effort to do things. It's like a car getting better mileage after a tune-up.

blood pressure

Blood pressure is better controlled in people with high blood pressure who exercise regularly. People who exercise regularly also tend to be more careful about diet and other health habits, which helps lower blood pressure.

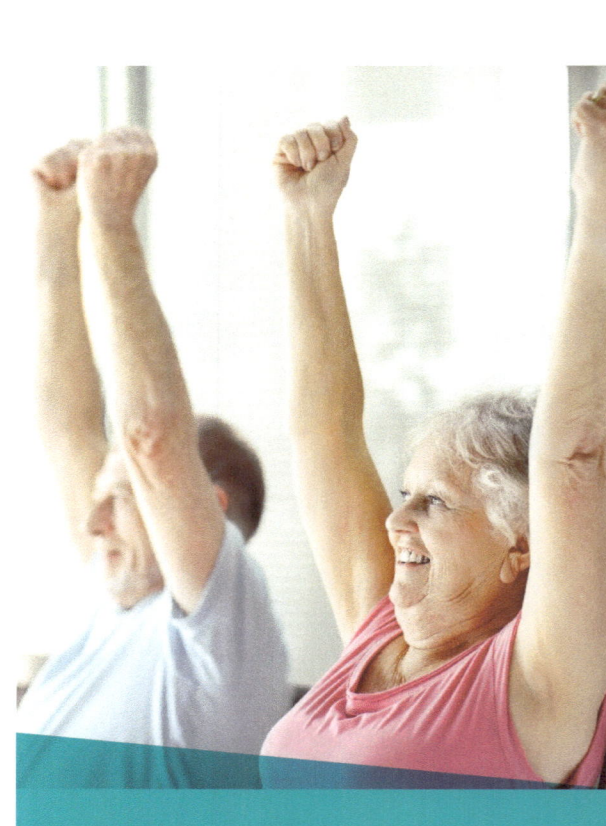

exercise can

help lower

blood pressure

body fat & weight loss

Too much body fat is not healthy. It not only makes the heart work harder, it also has been linked to other health problems. Fat around the waist is more dangerous than fat around the hips, but all fat is bad. Exercise and diet are two ways to lose body fat and weight. For every 3,500 calories you either don't eat or use up with activity, your weight goes down one pound. So if you ate 250 fewer calories a day and used up 250 more calories a day in exercise, it would take 7 days to lose one pound.

As you exercise, your body muscle mass will increase and your body fat will decrease. Since muscle weighs more than fat, the scales might not show your true improvement right away. You may want to get your body fat and muscle measured. You can also use the Body Mass Index (BMI) chart on page 9 to tell if your weight is in a healthy range.

Another way to judge body fat is your waist size. Your waist size is way too large if it is:

- 35 inches or more for women

- 40 inches or more
  for men

Measure your waist straight around at the top of your hip bone.

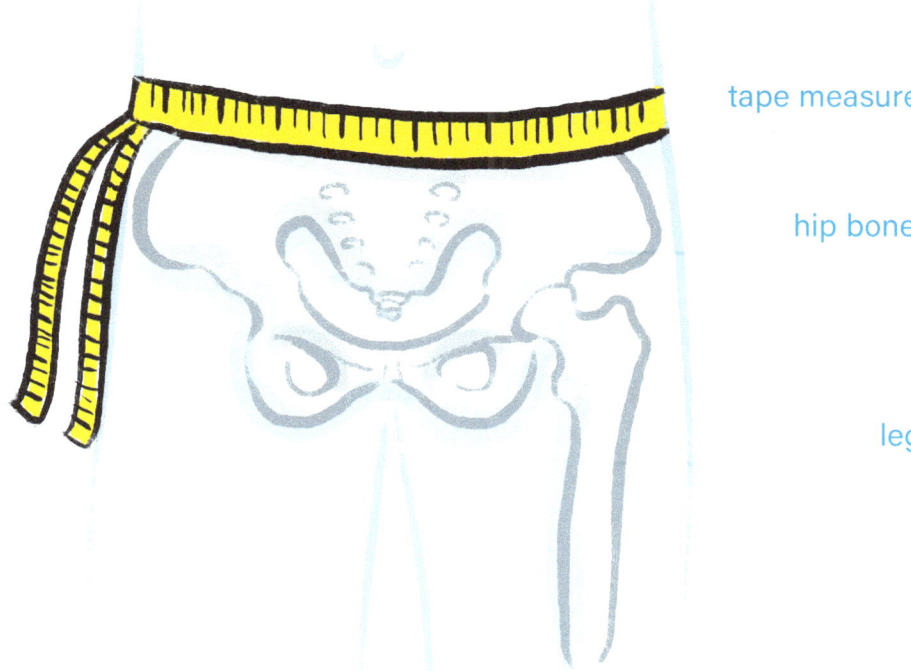

tape measure

hip bone

leg

Calories burned per hour

Count calories burned with exercise. Here is what to expect.

ACTIVITY	CALORIES burned/hour
calisthenics (fast pace)	600
cycling (outdoors, 13 mph)	660
dancing (fast pace, modern)	360
handball	660
pitching	450
rope skipping (easy pace)	300
rope skipping (fast pace)	800
rowing machine	840
running (5.5 mph)	675
running (7 mph)	870
skating (easy pace)	420
skiing (downhill, fast)	600
skiing (Nordic, 5 mph)	700
softball	280
stationary cycling (moderate)	450
swimming (crawl)	750
tennis (singles)	480
volleyball (competitive)	450
walking or slow jogging (4.5 mph)	450

Burning 2,000 or more calories a week in aerobic exercise lowers your risk for heart and blood vessel disease. Walking or jogging 1 mile can burn 100 calories. 2000 calories would take about 20 miles. You do get health benefits if you exercise less.

Body mass index (BMI)*

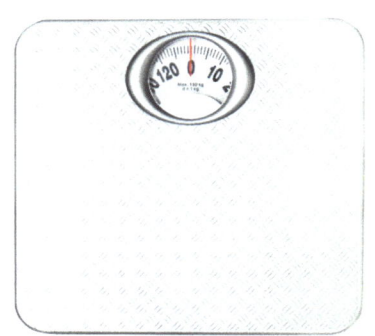

Here is how to use this body mass index (BMI) chart. If your BMI score is:

- **less than 25,** you are in a **healthy weight** range

- **between 25 and 30,** you are **overweight**

- **30 or higher,** you are considered **obese**

To use this chart, find your height in inches on the left side of the chart (Example: 5 feet = 60 inches). Then move across that row to find your weight (Example: 123 pounds). Move to the top of your weight column and look at the number. Your BMI score is 24.

Your BMI score is:

Your Height (inches)	19	20	21	22	23	24	25	26	27	28	29	30	31	32	33	34	35
	Your Weight (pounds)																
58"	91	96	100	105	110	115	119	124	129	134	138	143	148	153	158	162	167
59"	94	99	104	109	114	119	124	128	133	138	143	148	153	158	163	168	173
60" (EXAMPLE:)	97	102	107	112	118	123	128	133	138	143	148	153	158	163	168	174	179
61"	100	106	111	116	122	127	132	137	143	148	153	158	164	169	174	180	185
62"	104	109	115	120	126	131	136	142	147	153	158	164	169	175	180	186	191
63"	107	113	118	124	130	135	141	146	152	158	163	169	175	180	186	191	197
64"	110	116	122	128	134	140	145	151	157	163	169	174	180	186	192	197	204
65"	114	120	126	132	138	144	150	156	162	168	174	180	186	192	198	204	210
66"	118	124	130	136	142	148	155	161	167	173	179	186	192	198	204	210	216
67"	121	127	134	140	146	153	159	166	172	178	185	191	198	204	211	217	223
68"	125	131	138	144	151	158	164	171	177	184	190	197	203	210	216	223	230
69"	128	135	142	149	155	162	169	176	182	189	196	203	209	216	223	230	236
70"	132	139	146	153	160	167	174	181	188	195	202	209	216	222	229	236	243
71"	136	143	150	157	165	172	179	186	193	200	208	215	222	229	236	243	250
72"	140	147	154	162	169	177	184	191	199	206	213	221	228	235	242	250	258
73"	144	151	159	166	174	182	189	197	204	212	219	227	235	242	250	257	265
74"	148	155	163	171	179	186	194	202	210	218	225	233	241	249	256	264	272
75"	152	160	168	176	184	192	200	208	216	224	232	240	248	256	264	272	279
76"	156	164	172	180	189	197	205	213	221	230	238	246	254	263	271	279	287

*From the National Heart, Lung and Blood Institute

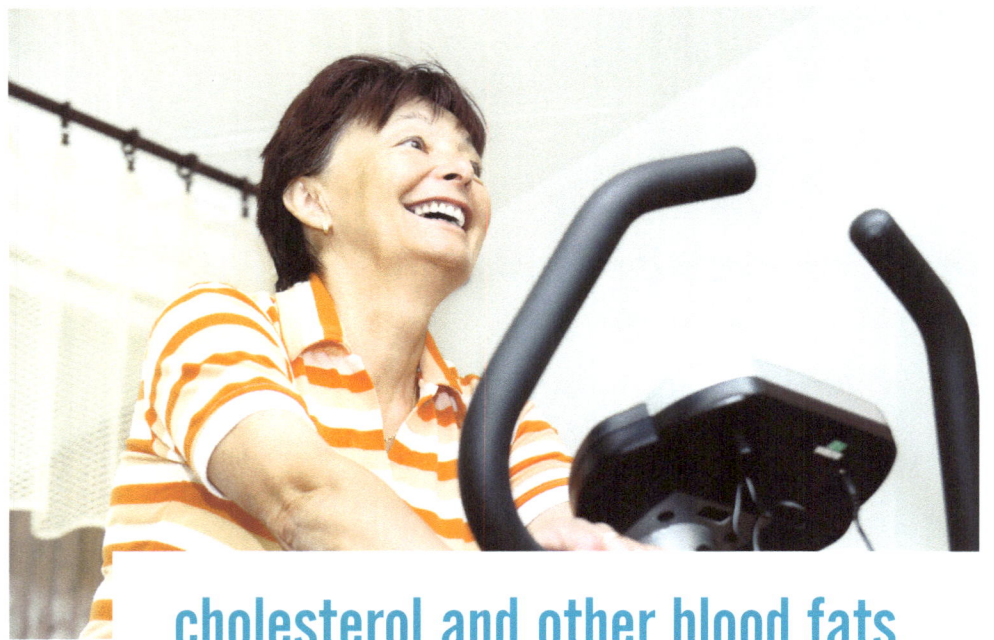

cholesterol and other blood fats

Cholesterol is a blood fat, and there are two ways you get it. Your body makes it, and it is in some foods. Your body has several types of cholesterol or blood fats. For example, **HDL cholesterol** is a **good** type of blood fat and **LDL cholesterol** and **triglycerides** are **bad** blood fats. Too little good and too much bad blood fat may cause blockage in the blood vessel walls and reduce blood flow. This raises your risk of a heart attack or damage to other parts of the body.

Exercise helps your body's HDL increase and triglycerides decrease. This is what you want since **low levels of HDL,** as well as **high levels of triglycerides,** have been **linked to heart disease.**

Ask your HCP what your numbers should be

total cholesterol below ▶

triglycerides ▶

LDL cholesterol ▶

HDL cholesterol ▶

Other changes in the blood

blood sugar (glucose)

Exercise helps a person control blood sugar and body weight. This, along with diet, is sometimes all that is needed to control type 2 diabetes. Regular exercise, along with diet, can also help those who take insulin. They may not be able to give up insulin, but they may not need to use as much to control blood sugar. See page 74 for more about diabetes and exercise.

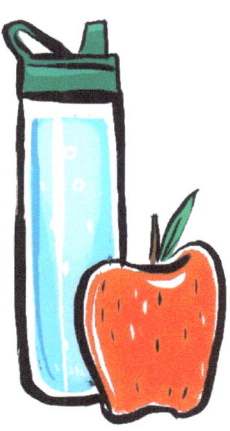

blood clotting

It is normal for blood to form clots and break them up. Platelets are the parts of blood that help make blood clots. In making these clots, the platelets become "sticky." They stick to each other and to the side of the blood vessel wall. This "sticking" together forms the blood clot. If the clot does not break up or dissolve, it may get bigger. This can harm the part of the body where it forms. For example, a blood clot in a blood vessel going to the heart muscle (coronary artery) may lead to a heart attack.

Exercise helps reduce platelet "stickiness" but not enough to make you bleed. This means there is less chance that harmful clots will form.

exercise helps to lower blood sugar and reduce the risk of blood clots

metabolic syndrome

You have metabolic syndrome if you have at least 3 of these 5 conditions:

waist in inches (see page 7 for how to measure)	40 or more for men 35 or more for women
blood pressure	higher than 120/80
blood triglycerides	above 150 mg/dL
HDL cholesterol in blood	less than 40 for men less than 50 for women
blood sugar	100 mg/dL or above

When you group these risk factors, you have a much greater chance of heart disease.

mental stress, depression, anxiety

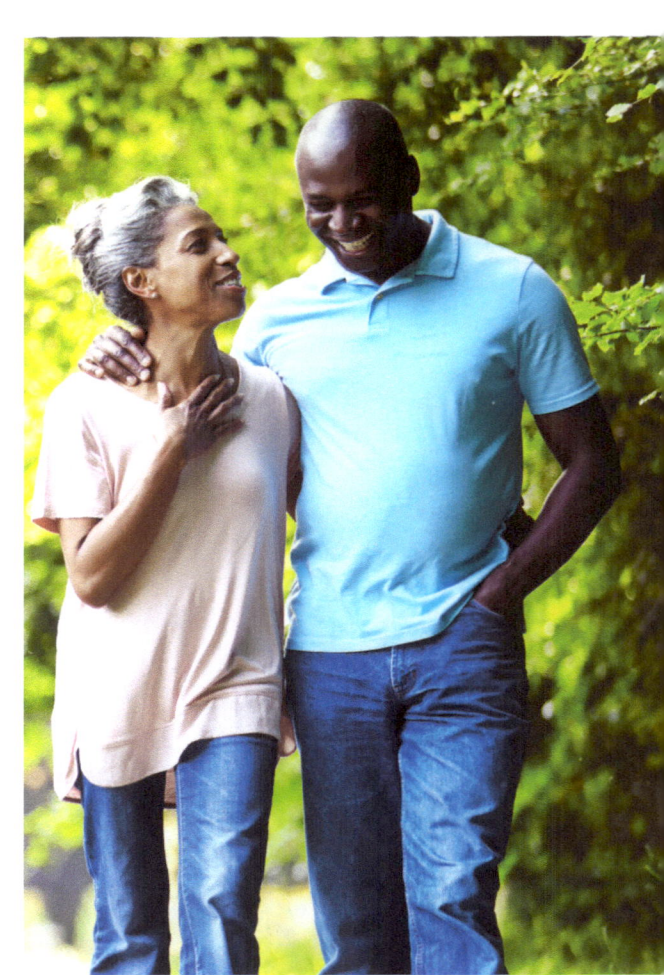

Exercise makes us feel better. **For a heart patient, exercise is a good way to control mental stress** and **prevent depression.** Feeling depressed or "blue" is less common in those who exercise regularly with such activities as walking, jogging, or playing tennis.

People who tend to be angry or hostile are at greater risk for heart disease. Exercise can reduce this risk. It lets a person work off some of the pressure and anxiety.

How to exercise

The 3 parts of a good exercise program include:

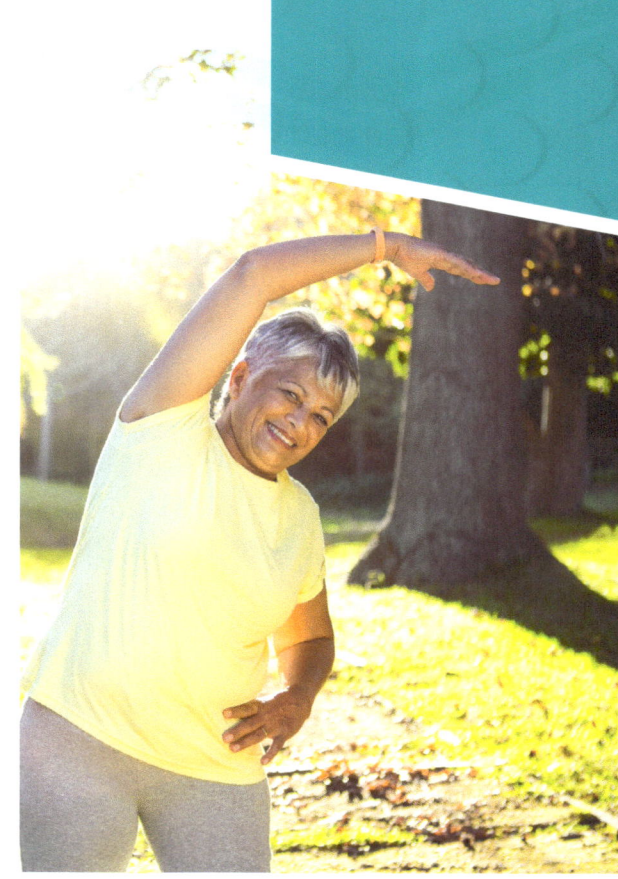

1. aerobic exercise (may be done all at once or broken into segments)

2. stretching and flexibility exercises (pgs 30-52)

3. strength or resistance training (see pgs 53-66)

It is best to warm up for 2-3 minutes before any exercise. The best warm up is one that uses the same muscles you use during your exercise.

Number 1, most of your exercise time should be spent in aerobic exercise. Aerobic exercise trains the heart muscle, helps the lungs take in more oxygen and helps your body in other ways (see page 5). Walking, jogging, cycling, dancing, swimming and cross-country skiing are examples of aerobic exercises. Sports that stop and go, like tennis, are less aerobic but are also good for training the heart.

Number 2, stretching and flexibility exercises should be done after aerobic exercise when the muscles are warm. This can help you avoid feeling stiff and sore later. Do these 3-4 times each week.

Number 3, strength or resistance training with weights or machines, should be done 2 to 3 times each week.

This is in addition to your aerobic exercise and stretching/flexibility exercises.

1. Aerobic exercise

Aerobic exercise is the most important part of exercise for your heart and health.

The harder you work, the more oxygen your body needs. After a few months of aerobic training, the heart can pump more blood and oxygen to the body with less effort. As a result, you will be able to better control blood pressure, blood fats, blood sugar, body fat and stress.

Aerobic exercise should be **done for a certain amount of time.** It is best if done for 30-60 minutes* for at least 5 times each week. Aerobic exercise can be done all at once or broken into segments. It is good to mix up your aerobic exercise routine. For example, change how hard you are exercising by going slow, then faster, then slower. But still exercise your full amount. If 30 minutes is hard to find, try doing 10 to 15 minutes 2-3 times a day.

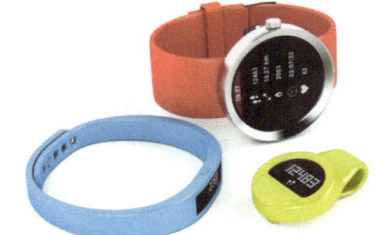

A pedometer can be used to help you see how much walking you do at work or at other times during the day. Many pedometers include a free app for your phone or tablet that helps you track your activity and meals. It is good to walk up to 10,000 steps a day.

Aerobic exercise not only brings oxygen to the heart and muscles, it also burns calories. For these reasons, aerobic exercises are talked about in terms of oxygen used (METS) or calories burned. You will find tables showing the MET (metabolic) level (page 16) or calories burned (page 8) for some favorite activities. A good rule to remember is that brisk walking or jogging 1 mile burns about 100 calories.

Before and after any aerobic exercise you should warm up and cool down. Examples of warm up and cool down are:

- walk slowly for 200 to 400 feet

- pedal a bike slowly for 3–5 minutes with no resistance

If you just stop after your aerobic workout, the muscles tend to get stiff, and blood tends to pool in the veins. This could cause you to get light-headed or even faint.

*30 minutes of aerobic exercise does not include your time for stretching and flexibility. Make sure to add time for these.

Metabolic Equivalents (METS)

One way to decide how much exercise to do is to use METS (metabolic equivalents). One MET is how much oxygen the body needs while sitting quietly and doing nothing. An activity that uses four times as much oxygen is equal to a 4 MET level. Five times as much oxygen equals 5 METS and so on.

It does not matter how long you do the activity. The MET level stays the same as long as you do not change how fast or how hard you work out. For example, you can walk at a 15 minute per mile pace for 3 minutes or 30 minutes and still be at a 4 to 5 MET level.

The MET level you choose depends on the condition of your heart and health. As you train, you will be able to work at higher levels. See examples of MET levels on next page

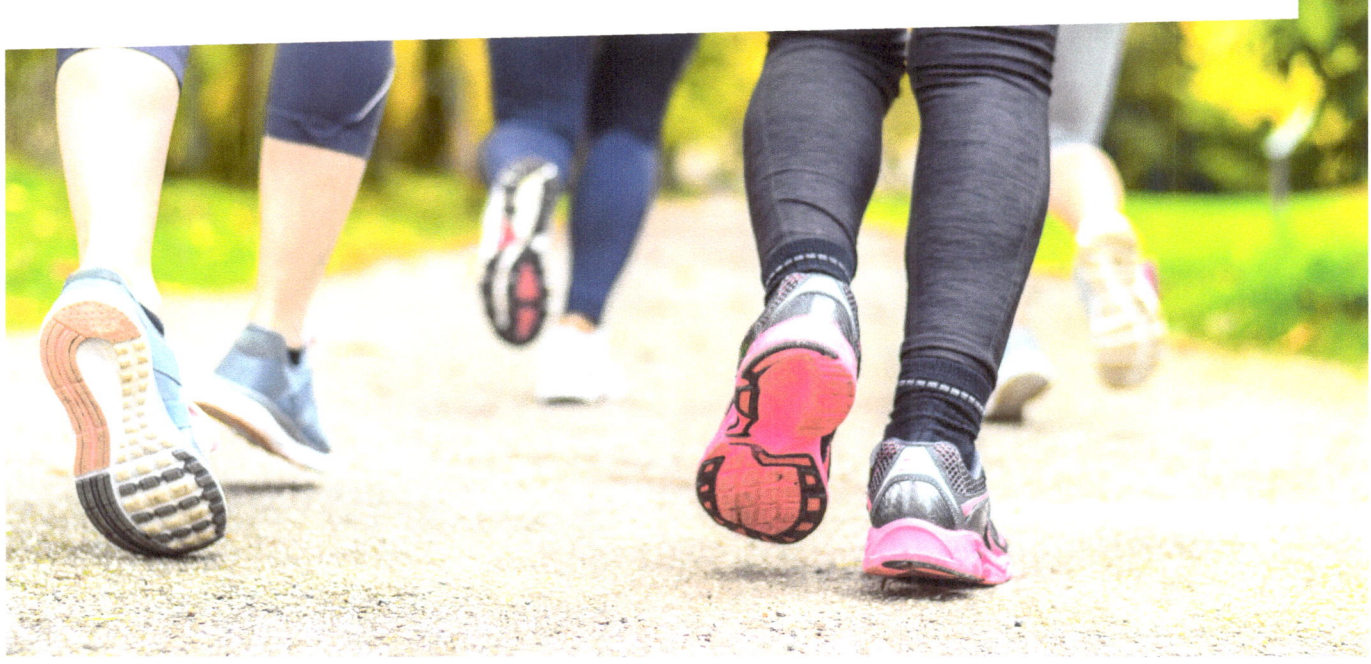

You do not need to exercise at the same MET level for a full 30 to 60 minutes. You can cycle at 10 mph (5–6 METS) for 15 minutes and jog at a 12 minute per mile pace (8 METS) for 15 minutes. The goal is simply to achieve your aerobic workout of 30-60 minutes, whether at different MET levels or the same.

The higher the MET level, the better conditioned your body will be.

Sample Play Activities
Grouped by intensitiy

ACTIVITIES	METS	ACTIVITIES	METS
MILD		**HARD**	
billiards (pool)	2.4	chopping wood	4.9
canoeing (slowly)	2.5	climbing hills (no load)	6.9
dancing (ballroom, slow)	2.9	climbing hills (11 lb load)	7.4
golf (with cart)	2.5	cycling (moderately, about 10 mph)	5.7
horseback riding (walking)	2.3	dancing:	
playing a musical instrument:		aerobic or ballet	6.0
accordion	1.8	ballroom (fast) or square	5.5
cello	2.3	jogging (10 minute mile)	10.2
flute	2.5	rope skipping	12.0
piano	2.3	skating:	
violin	2.5	ice	5.5
volleyball (non-competitive)	2.9	roller	6.5
walking (30 minute mile)	2.5	skiing (water or downhill)	6.8
MODERATE		squash	12.1
calisthenics (no weight)	4.0	surfing	6.0
cycling (slowly, about 5-6 mph)	3.5	swimming	7.0
golf (without cart)	4.4	tennis (doubles)	5.0
swimming (slow)	4.5	jogging (12 minute mile)	8.0
walking (20 minute mile)	3.3		
walking (15 minute mile)	4.5		

Daily Living Activities

ACTIVITIES	METS	ACTIVITIES	METS
gardening (no lifting)	4.4	riding in a car, truck, etc.	1.0
household tasks (moderate)	3.5	sitting, light activity	1.5
lifting items (continuously)	4.0	taking out trash	3.0
loading/unloading car	3.0	vacuuming	3.5
lying quietly	1.0	walking the dog	3.0
mopping	3.5	walking from house to car or bus	2.5
mowing lawn (power mower)	4.5	watering plants	2.5
raking lawn	4.0		

Adapted from AHA Exercise Standards

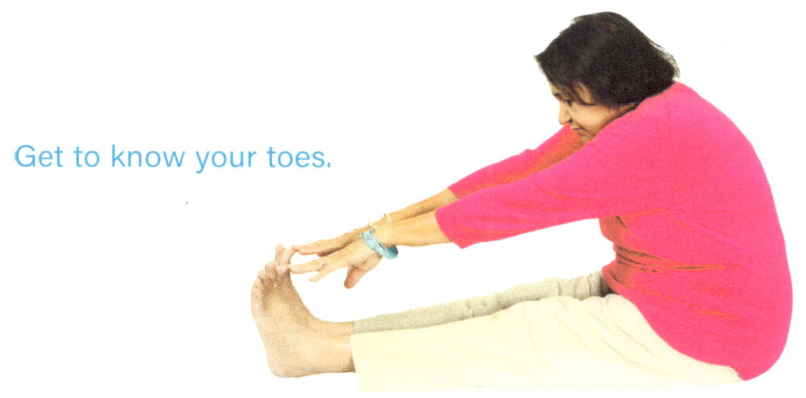

Get to know your toes.

2. Stretching and flexibility exercises*

Some exercises will help you stretch and flex your muscles. These exercises should be done after your aerobic exercise when muscles are warm. Do them 3-4 times each week. They can be light stretches and other exercises. How long you do each exercise depends on what you will be doing later and for how long. This can be planned with your HCP.

The best reason to stretch and tone the muscles is to stay flexible. When you are flexible, or loose, your muscles and joints can bend and move more easily with each exercise. This can help prevent injuries.

Another reason to stretch and warm up the muscles is to improve the blood supply to them. Blood vessels in a warm, loose muscle are better able to take oxygen to the muscle and remove waste products from it.

There are many reasons why people are not flexible. Some are age, medical conditions such as arthritis, lack of exercise, cold weather or body fat. Others are bone structure and the amount of muscle around the bones. Even some aerobic exercise can make you less flexible, but this can be overcome with stretching and flexibility exercise.

Other activities like pilates and Tai Chi can help muscle strength and flexibility. These also help with balance and make your aerobic exercise easier.

Not doing stretching and flexibility exercises can lead to sore tendons (tendinitis), inflamed joints (bursitis) and muscle strain. If you already have one of these problems, ask your HCP which exercises are best for you.

* 30 minutes of aerobic exercise does not include your time for stretching and flexibility. Make sure to add time for these.

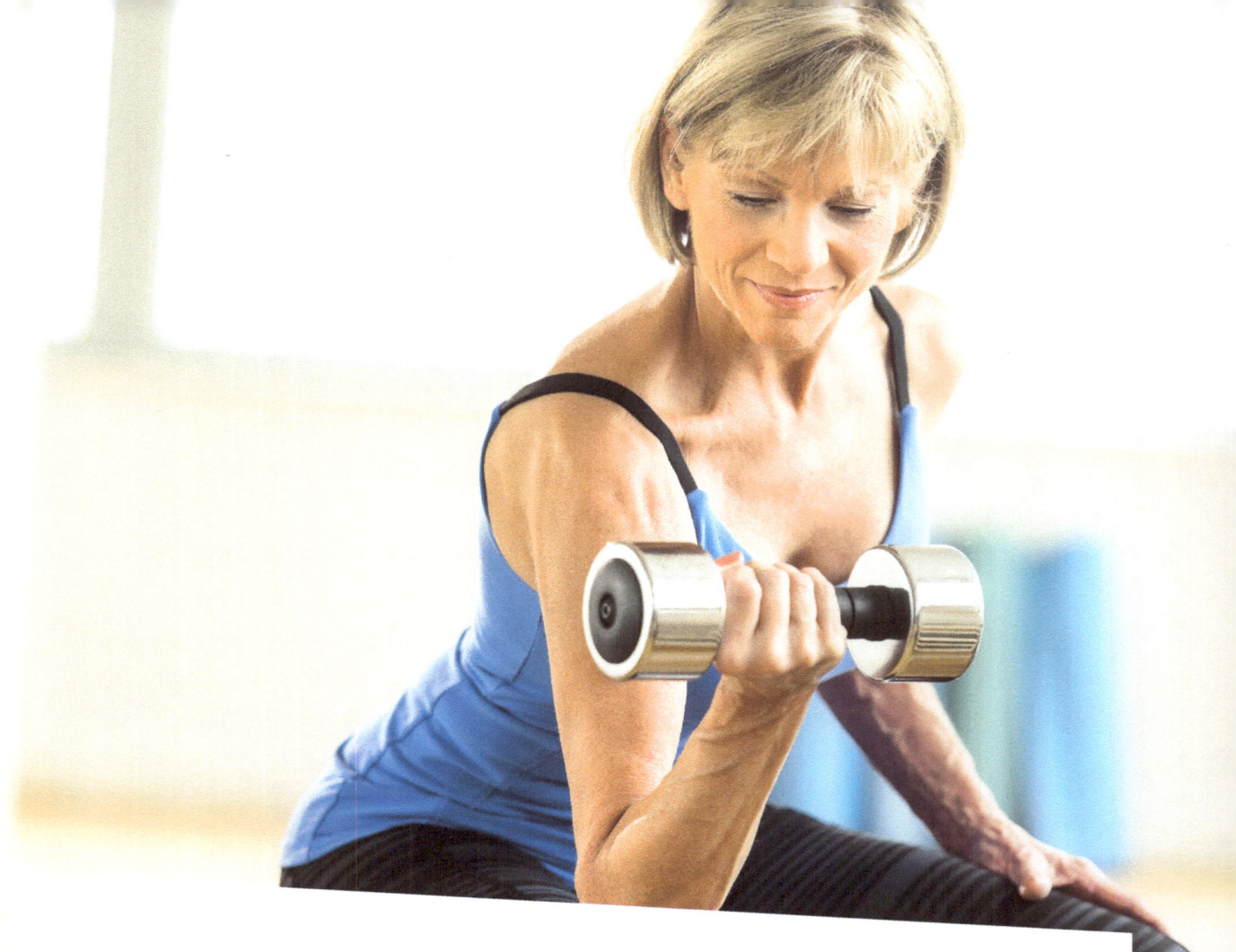

3. Strength or resistance exercise training

You gain strength in many ways. The best ways are to lift weights, do push-ups and work out with equipment made for building strength. Low to moderate level strength training is safe for people with heart disease, but check it out with your HCP before starting.

Muscles tend to get smaller and weaker as we age. But weight lifting is a very good way for both men and women to keep their muscles strong. You can use dumbbells, barbells and ankle and wrist weights for building strength.

It does not matter if you lift weights before or after aerobic exercise. A good plan is 2 to 3 days a week. Muscles need to rest between times of weight or strength training.

How hard to exercise

To exercise safely, you need to know how hard to exercise. This is true whether you have a heart condition or are healthy. You can learn by counting your pulse for your target heart rate or by tuning in to how you feel or how hard you are exercising (perceived exertion).

your pulse and target heart rates

Everyone has a **peak heart rate** and a **target heart rate range.** Your peak heart rate is how fast your heart can beat at the end of an exercise test or at exhaustion. It is not the heart rate at which you exercise when working out on your own. For your own workouts, you will want to know your target heart rate range. This will be somewhere between 50% and 85% of the peak rate you reached on your exercise test. **People with heart problems** should have their HCP tell them their target **exercise heart rate range.**

Your target heart rate range can be found in different ways. The exact and safe way to find your target heart rate is through an **exercise stress test.**

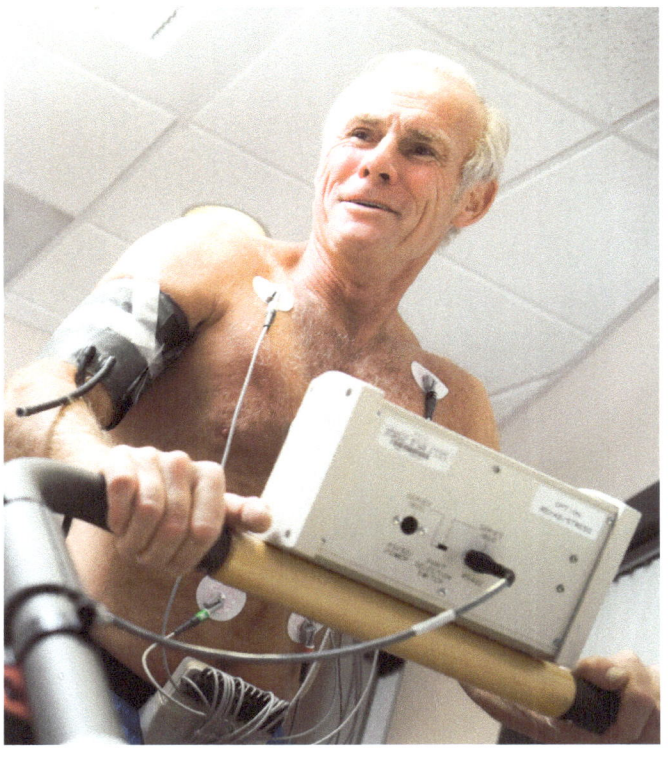

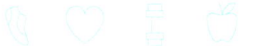

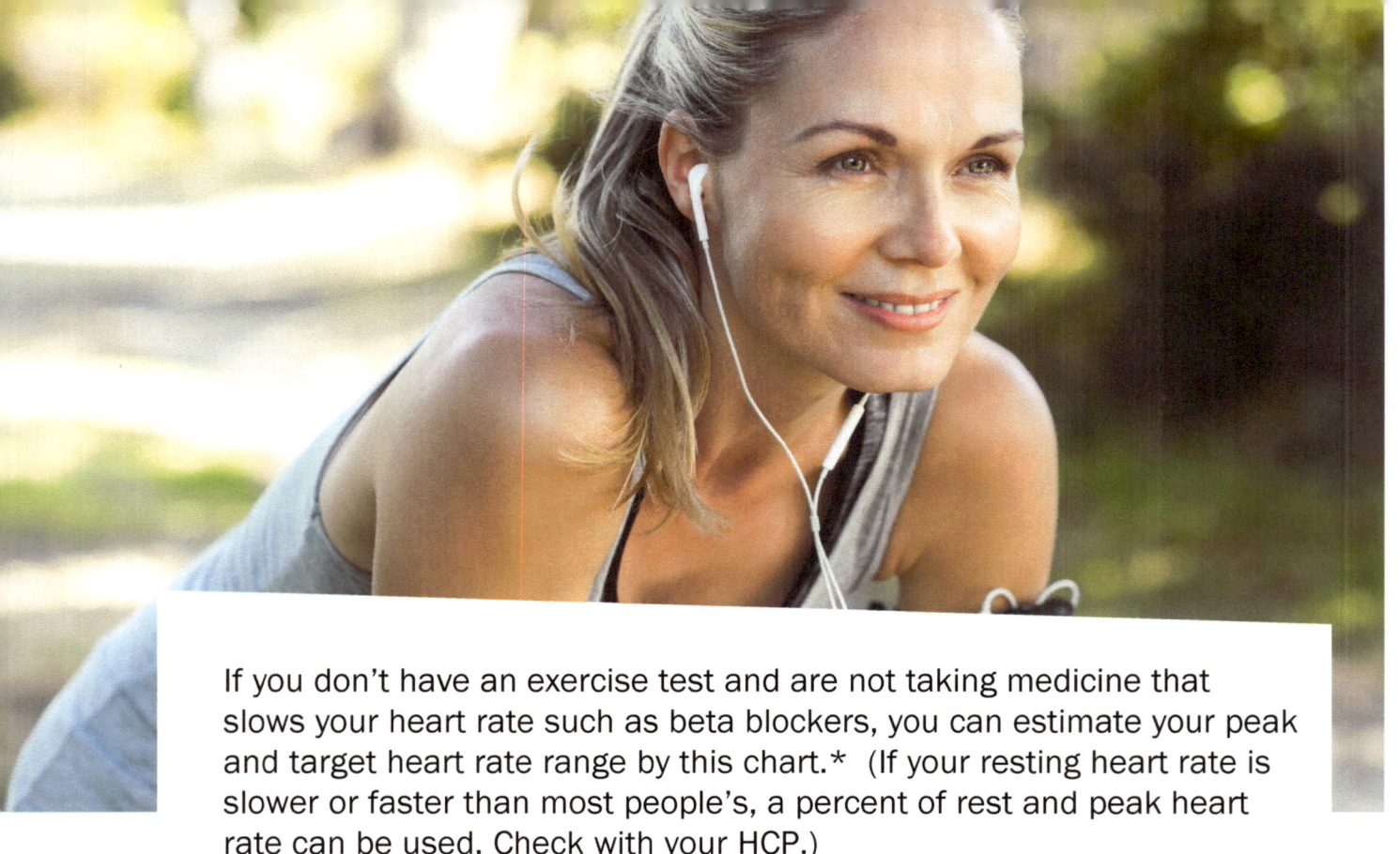

If you don't have an exercise test and are not taking medicine that slows your heart rate such as beta blockers, you can estimate your peak and target heart rate range by this chart.* (If your resting heart rate is slower or faster than most people's, a percent of rest and peak heart rate can be used. Check with your HCP.)

Age		20	25	30	35	40	45	50	55	60	65	70	75	80	85	90
Peak Heart Rates		197	195	193	191	189	187	184	182	180	178	176	174	172	170	168
Target Heart Rates	85%	167	166	164	162	161	159	156	155	153	151	150	148	146	144	143
	75%	148	146	145	143	142	140	138	136	135	133	132	130	129	127	126
	60%	118	117	116	115	113	112	110	109	108	107	106	104	103	102	101
	50%	99	98	97	96	95	94	92	91	90	89	88	87	86	85	84

Data based on that of Sheffield, et al, and Pollock and Wilmore.

If you are just beginning your exercise program or you have not exercised in some time, your target heart rate should be in the 50% to 60% range. After about 4 to 6 weeks, you may want to increase your level or you may want to stay at your same target heart rate range. If you choose to increase, do so slowly. Work out at the 60% to 75% level until you are comfortable before going to the 75% to 85% range. Your goal is to find the target heart rate range at which you can exercise with comfort—whether it is 50%, 75% or 85%.

*People on certain medicines, such as beta blockers, may have lower heart rate ranges than those in this chart. If this applies to you, ask your HCP for your target heart rate.

Count your pulse to see if you are exercising at your target heart rate. If you don't reach your target range, you may not be doing enough exercise. If you go over it, you may be doing too much.

This is what to do:

- As soon as you stop exercising, find your pulse at your wrist.

- Count it for 10 seconds.

- Multiply what you count by 6. This will be your one minute heart rate at that time.

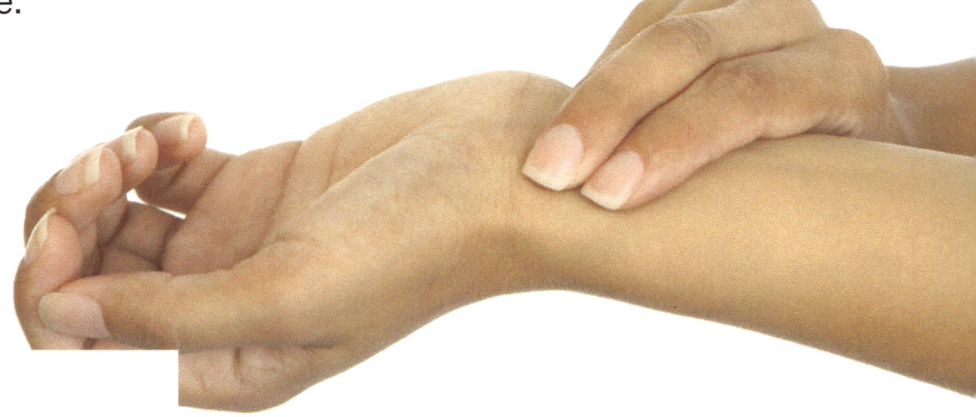

Example:

10 second count	=	20
multiply		x 6
1 minute heart rate		120

What you get should match your target heart rate range. If you get a heart rate of 160 but your target heart rate range is 94 to 145, you are working too hard. If you get only 90, most likely you are not exercising hard enough. If what you calculate never matches your target heart rate range, talk to your HCP. Either the target rates should be changed or you should do more or less exercise.

tuning in to how you feel

Many people exercise by how hard they feel the exercise is or how hard they think they are working. This is called the rate of perceived exertion or RPE scale. The scale goes from 6 to 20 with 7 being very, very light work and 19 being very, very hard work.

To use this scale, you have to think about how hard you are working in terms of your level of fatigue, any shortness of breath and muscle or skeletal pain or aching. When you "average" all these feelings during your workout, your exercise should feel between fairly light work (11) and hard work (15). This 11 to 15 range is like working out at 50 to 85% of your peak heart rate. Remember, never go to exhaustion (19 or 20).

Some people like to use the 10 point Borg scale where 1 is very light and 10 is very, very hard. With this scale, you should exercise between 2 (fairly light) and 5 (hard).

THE BORG RPE SCALE

6
7...........................very, very light
8
9 ....very light
10
11 ....fairly light
12
13....................... somewhat hard
14
15...hard
16
17....................................very hard
18
19.........................very, very hard
20

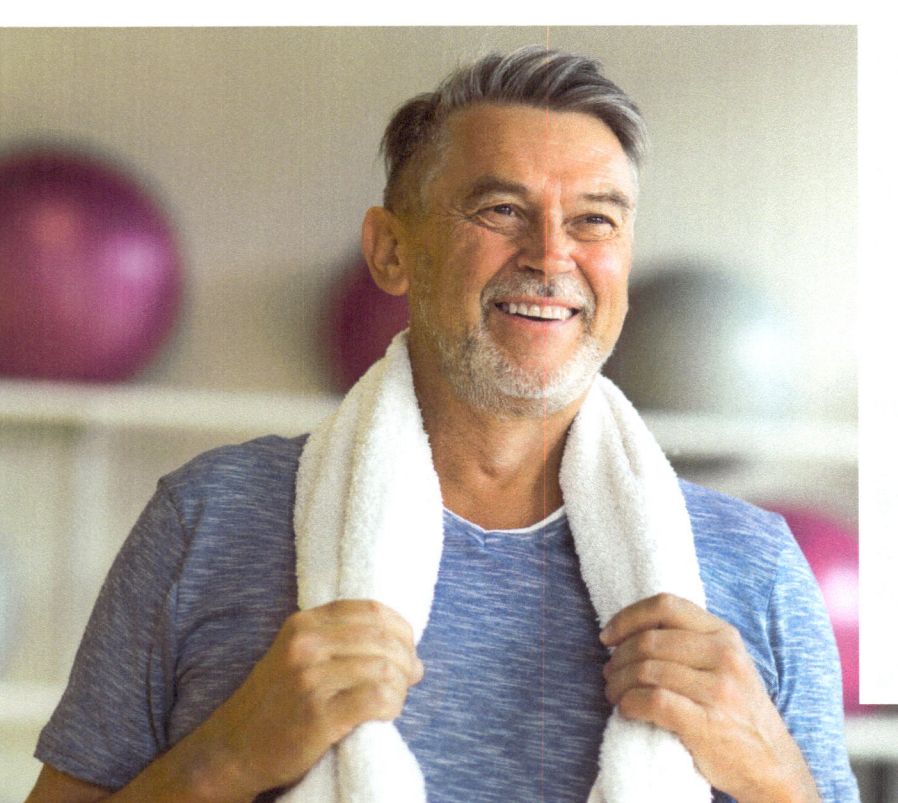

Guidelines for people with a heart condition*

Jogging (running)	Best to do in a medically supervised program. If done on your own, use a lower target heart rate.
Brisk Walking	Very good training. May be done alone or with others.
Swimming	Lower your target heart rate by 10 beats/minute since you may not notice your heart problem while swimming. Do not swim in very cold water.
Tennis	Doubles is less work for your heart than singles. Work up to singles.
Water Activities	Check with your HCP before water skiing or water activities as these may have bad effects on your blood pressure, heart rate or rhythm.
Snow Skiing	OK for some heart patients. Stay at moderate altitudes. Dress warmly. Wear layers that are insulated rather than heavy clothes. If taking beta blocker medicine, cold weather may cause numbness, tingling and discomfort in your hands and feet.
Stationary Bike	Excellent. No problems with weather. If you sweat while pedaling, use a fan to cool the body. (See pages 28–29.)
Biking Outdoors	Popular. Think about the weather before going out. Know when to turn around so you can return home before tiring.

*These are for aerobic exercises.

BEGINNERS & HEART PATIENTS, START HERE

warm up: 3 to 5 minutes of

- stretching/flexibility exercises (select 2 to 3 exercises)
- slow walking or cycling

workout: 20–30 minutes of aerobic exercise at the lower range of your target heart rate (50–60%) and rate of perceived exertion of 11–12 (take breaks as needed, but do a total of 20–30 minutes of exercise)

cool-down: 3 to 5 minutes of

- slow walking or cycling

Do this exercise program 5 to 6 days per week. Follow this routine for 2 or more weeks before going to the mid-level program. (You may choose to stay longer at this level.)

MID-LEVEL PROGRAM

warm up: 3 to 5 minutes of

- stretching/flexibility exercises (select 3 to 4 exercises)
- slowly start your aerobic exercise

workout: 30 to 45 minutes of aerobic exercise at the low to middle range of your target heart rate (60–70%) and perceived exertion range of 12–13

cool-down: 3 to 5 minutes of

- your slow aerobic exercises

Continue this exercise program 5 to 6 days per week. Follow this routine for 2 or more weeks before going to the advanced program. (You may choose to stay at this level.)

ADVANCED-LEVEL PROGRAM

warm up: 3 to 5 minutes of

- stretching/flexibility exercises (select 3 to 4 exercises)
- slowly start your aerobic exercise

workout: 30 to 60 minutes of aerobic exercise at the mid to upper range of your target heart rate (70–85%) and perceived exertion range of 13–15

cool-down: 5 minutes of

- your slow aerobic exercises

Continue this routine 5 to 6 days a week.

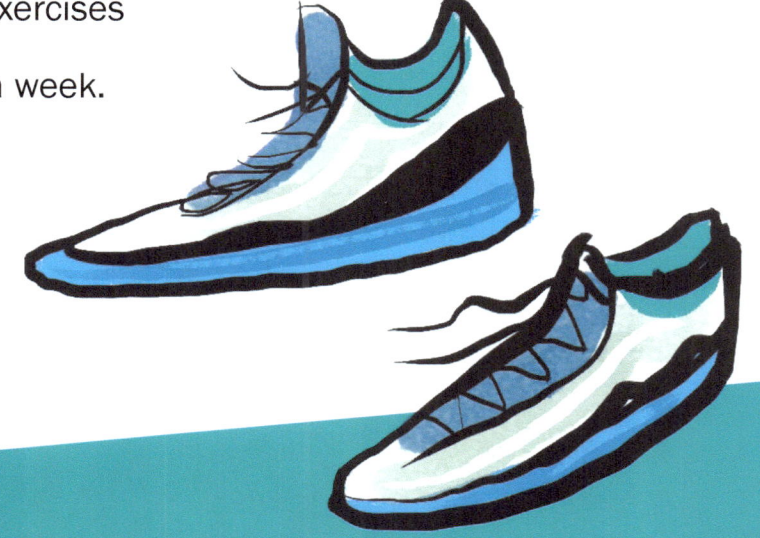

Never increase your exercise until the level you are on is easy for you to do and you aren't tired after a session. The least amount of time you should spend at each level is 2 weeks. People who are just starting to exercise and those who have medical conditions may want to stay longer at each level. Don't rush your exercise program. If you do, you could injure yourself. The most reward from exercise will come if you do it on a regular basis and if you are patient.

aerobic exercise programs

walking

The home-walk programs on this page and the next are for people with heart problems or beginners who want to start exercising. They help you start slowly and build endurance as you go.

You may not reach your target heart rate at first. This will happen as you work up to it with each week of exercise.

You should know the exact state of your health before starting either of these programs. Show these pages to your HCP and work out what's right for you.

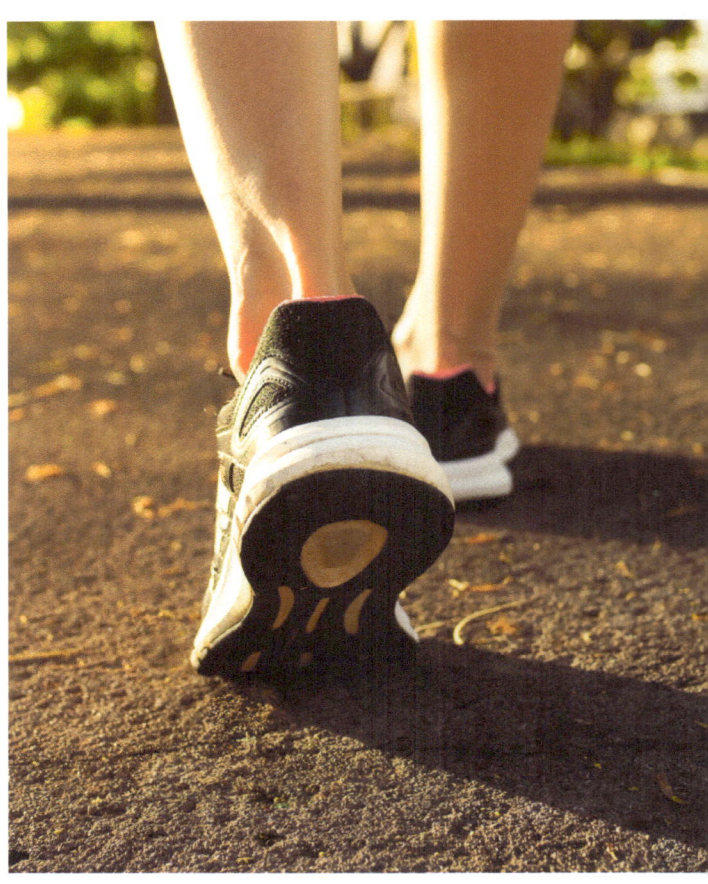

Easy Home-walk Program*			
WEEK	**DISTANCE**	**PACE**	**TIME**
Week 1	walk ½ mile twice a day	20 min/mile	10 minutes each time
Week 2	walk 1 mile/day	20 min/mile	20 minutes
Week 3	walk 1 ½ miles/day	20 min/mile	30 minutes
Week 4	walk 2 miles/day	20 min/mile	40 minutes
Week 5	walk 2 ½ miles/day	20 min/mile	50 minutes
Week 6-on	walk 3 miles/day	20 min/mile	60 minutes

*Check your pulse right after each walk. If your heart rate is higher than your target heart rate, do not go to the next week or level.

Harder Home-walk Program*

WEEK	DISTANCE	PACE	TIME
Week 1	walk ¾ mile twice a day	20 min/mile	15 minutes
Week 2	walk 1 mile/day	20 min/mile	20 minutes
Week 3	walk 1 ½ miles/day	18 min/mile	27 minutes
Week 4	walk 2 miles/day	17 min/mile	34 minutes
Week 5	walk 2 ½ miles/day	16 min/mile	40 minutes
Week 6	walk 3 miles/day	15 min/mile	45 minutes
Week 7	walk 3 ½ miles/day	15 min/mile	53 minutes
Week 8-on	walk 4 miles/day	14-15 min/mile	56-60 minutes

*Check your pulse right after each walk. If it is higher than your target heart rate, do not go to the next week or level.

**You may want to gradually increase your distance and keep your pace slower.

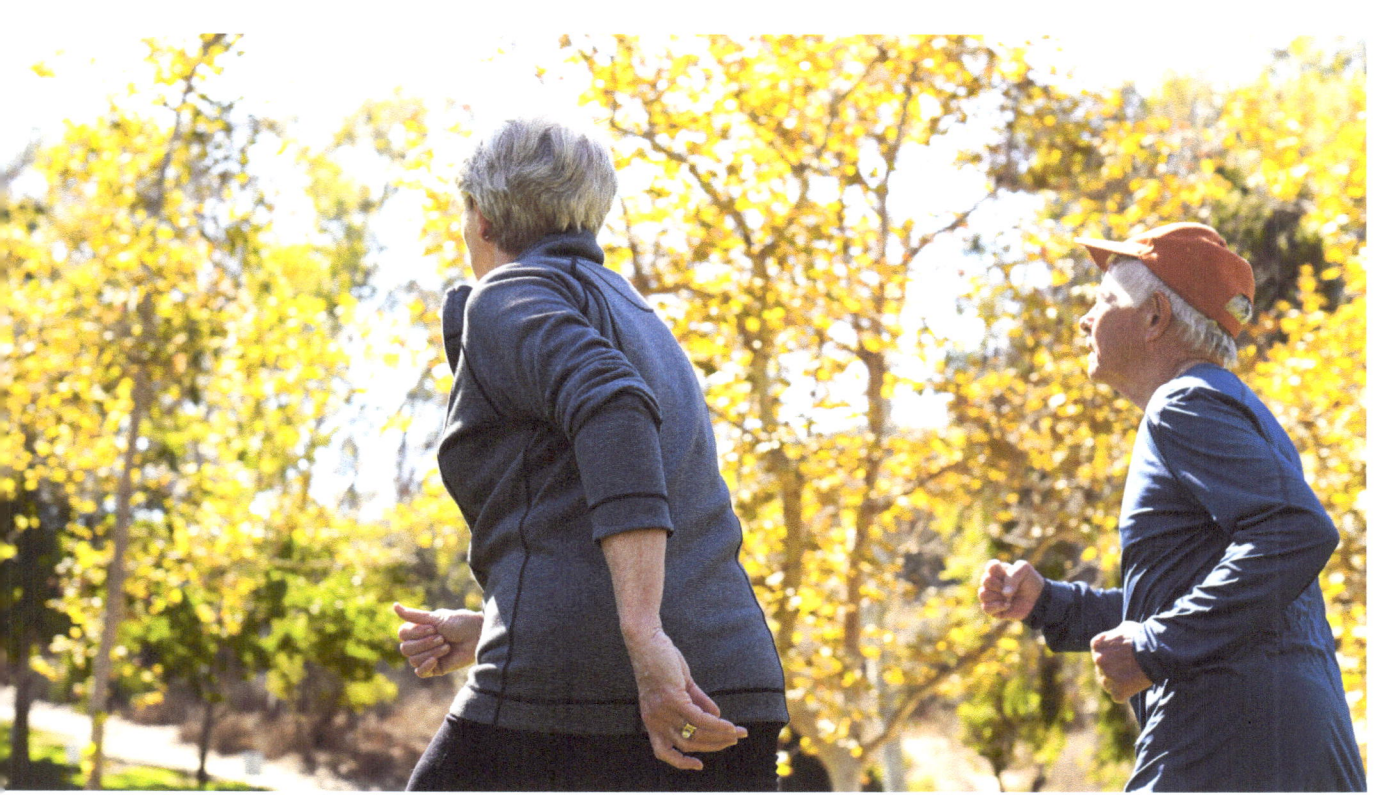

stationary bike

Many people like to exercise on a stationary bike. Bad weather, bad dogs and hills are no problem! You can also listen to music or watch TV while you exercise. Your exercise room should be a comfortable temperature and well ventilated.

Sit on the bike as shown here. Make sure your seat is comfortable and the right height. (See the picture below.)

Again, you may not reach your target heart rate at first. But you should be able to work up to it.

As with the home-walk programs, this is just a sample. Your exercise on a stationary bike may begin or end at a different level than someone else's. Find out what's right for you and stick to it.

Lean forward (a little). ▶

Relax body. ▶

Have a slight bend in the knee when pedal is closest to floor. ▶

Pedal on ball of foot. ▶

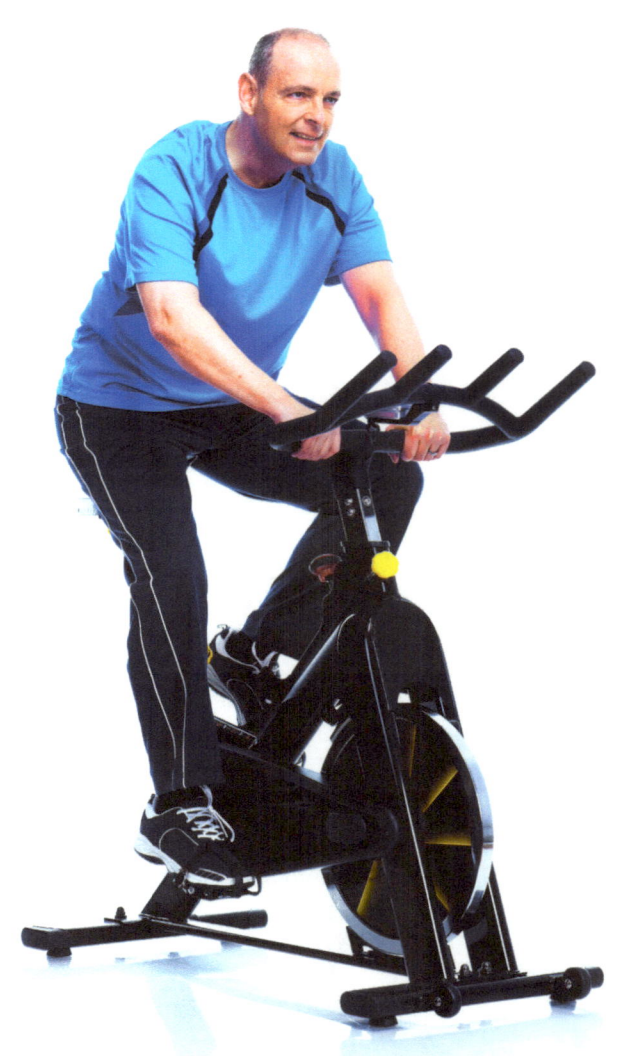

Stationary Bike Exercise Program

(for beginners and heart patients)

WEEK	TIME	SPEED	RESISTANCE
1	5 minutes pedaling 2 minutes resting 5 minutes pedaling	low	low
2	7 minutes pedaling 2 minutes resting 7 minutes pedaling	low	low
3	10 minutes pedaling 2 minutes resting 10 minutes pedaling	moderate	slight increase from week 2
4 and 5	2 minutes pedaling (warm-up) 20 minutes pedaling 2 minutes pedaling (cool-down)	low moderate low	low slight increase from week 3 low
6 and 7	2 minutes pedaling (warm-up) 25 minutes pedaling 2 minutes pedaling (cool-down)	low moderate low	low slight increase from week 5 low
8 and 9	2 minutes pedaling (warm-up) 30 minutes pedaling 2 minutes pedaling (cool-down)	low moderate to high low	low slight increase from week 7 low
10 and 11	2 minutes pedaling (warm-up) 35-40 minutes pedaling 2 minutes pedaling (cool-down)	low moderate to high low	low slight increase from week 9 low
12-on	2 minutes pedaling (warm-up) 40-60 minutes pedaling 2 minutes pedaling (cool-down)	low moderate to high low	low slight increase from week 11 low

Can be done on a bike that works both your arms and legs, or a bike that only works your legs.

To add resistance, adjust the tension on the bike so that it becomes harder to pedal. If you can't pedal at this higher level, don't stop. Lower the tension, and pedal for 1–2 minutes. When you feel better, adjust the tension back up slightly.

Do not add resistance if your Rate of Perceived Exertion exceeds 15 (or hard) or if your exercise heart rate is above your target level.

deep breaths

- Stand erect, with feet a short distance apart. Inhale as you lift your arms up.

- Exhale as you lower your arms.

- Repeat 2 times, slowly.

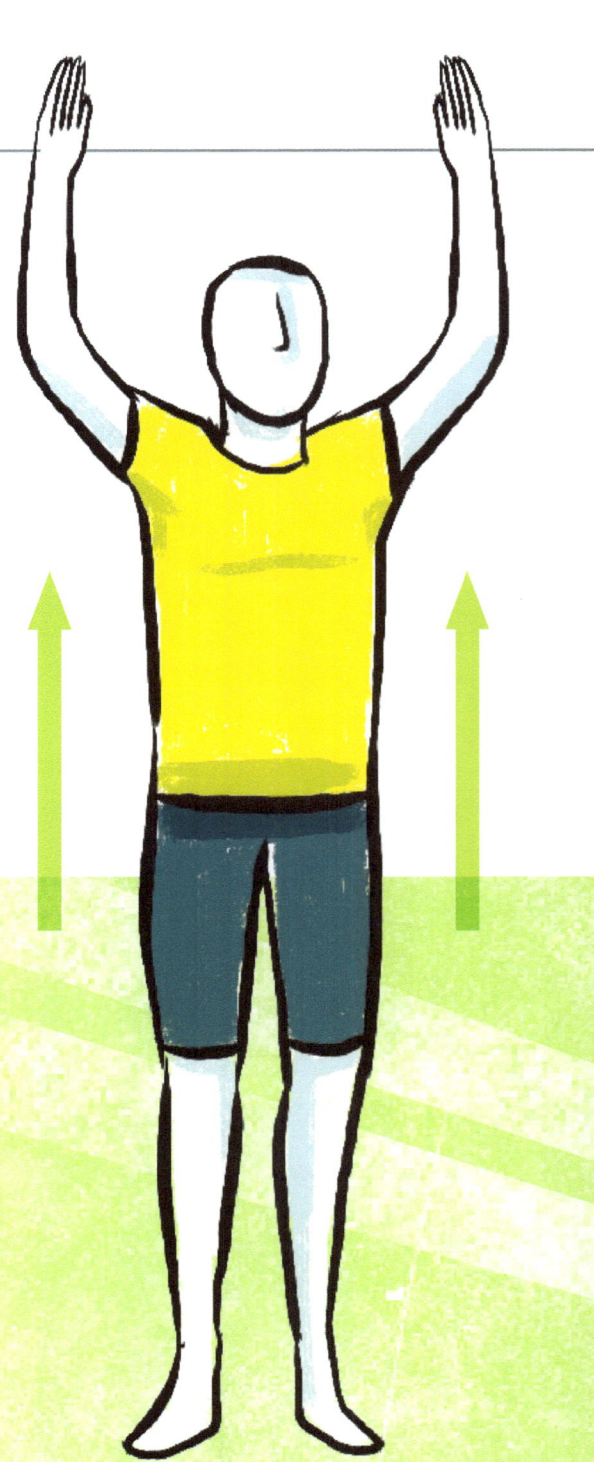

shoulder circles

- In a comfortable standing position, slowly shrug shoulders around in a circle 5 times.

- Then repeat going the other way.

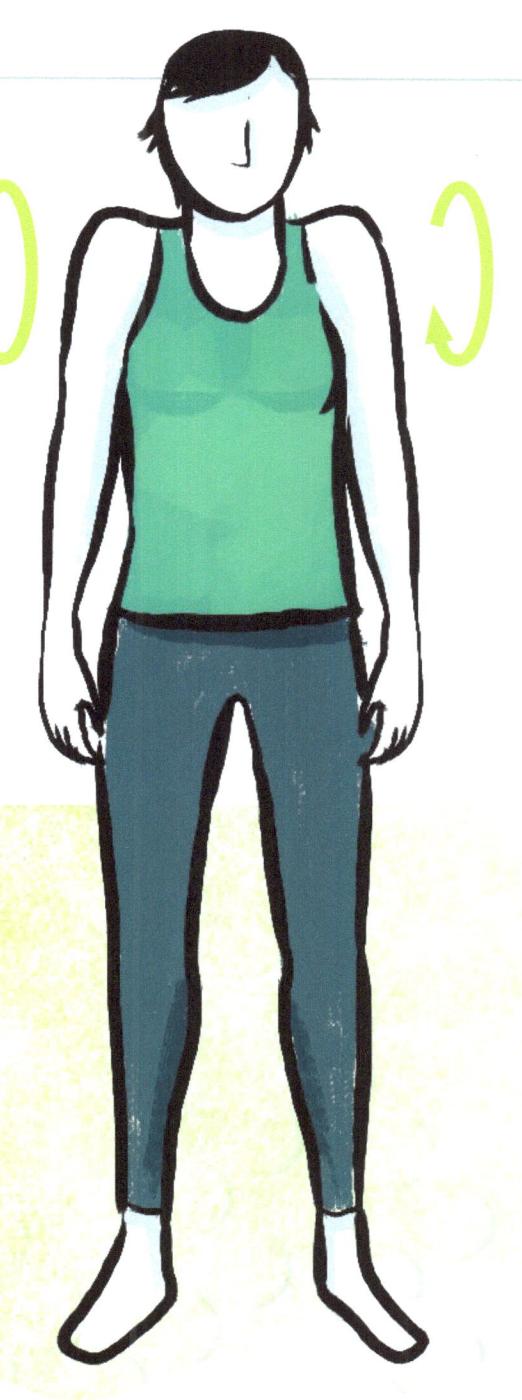

upper body side stretch

- Stand tall with feet apart 18 to 20 inches.

- Reach up with one arm and down with the other without bending forward or backward.

- Hold for 5 seconds. Switch arms.

- Repeat 2 times with each arm.

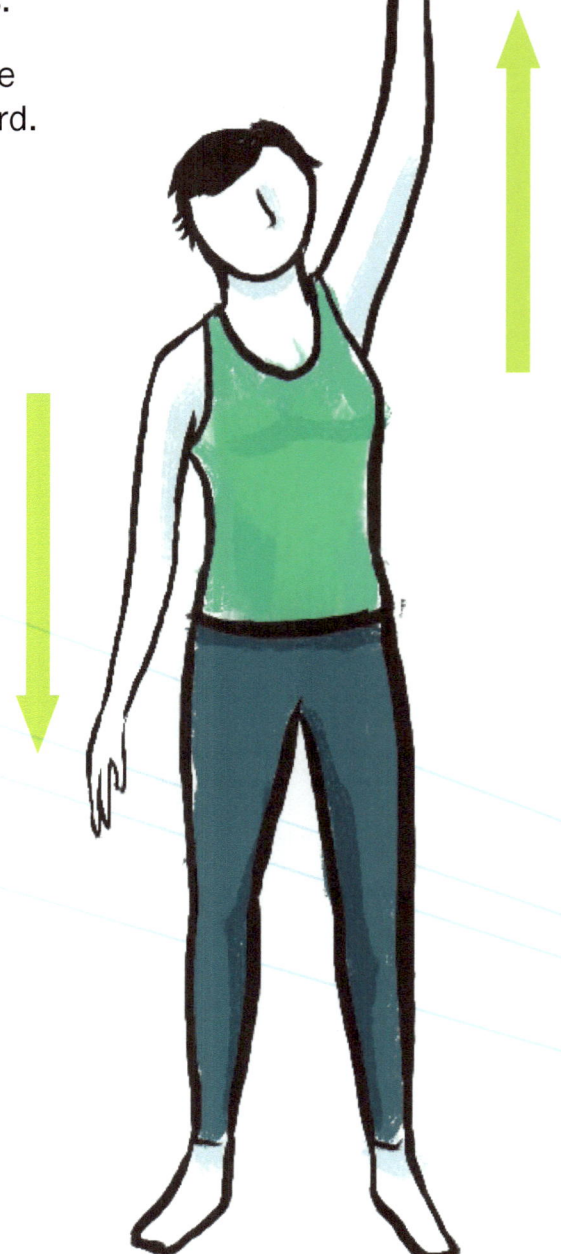

inner thigh stretch

- Face forward with feet in a wide stride (36 to 48 inches).

- Bend right knee over right foot, keeping left leg straight. Hold for 20 to 30 seconds. Then do the other side.

- Repeat 2 times.

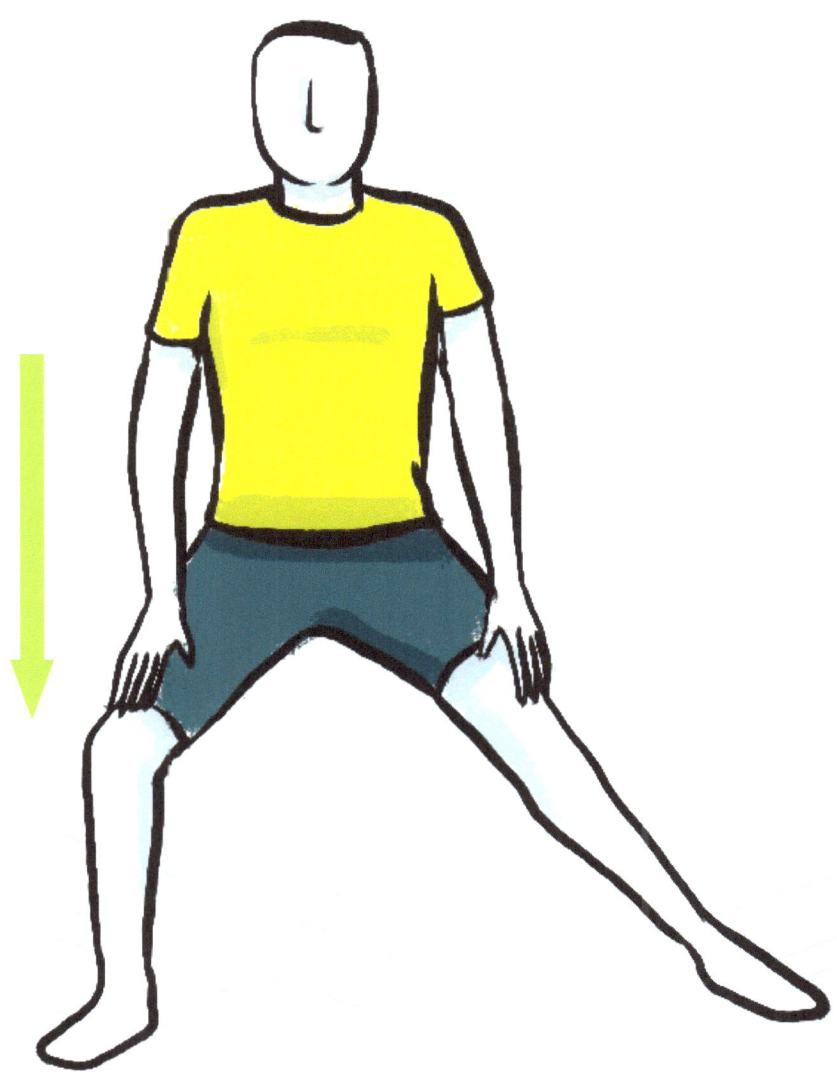

calf stretch

- Stand facing a wall with one leg in front of the other.

- Slightly bend front knee while keeping the back leg straight and pressing the back heel toward floor. Lean forward slightly toward wall while balancing with your hands on the wall. Keep your body in a straight line from your shoulders to your back heel. Hold position for 20 to 30 seconds. Return to starting position. Repeat exercise with other leg in back.

- Repeat 2 times.

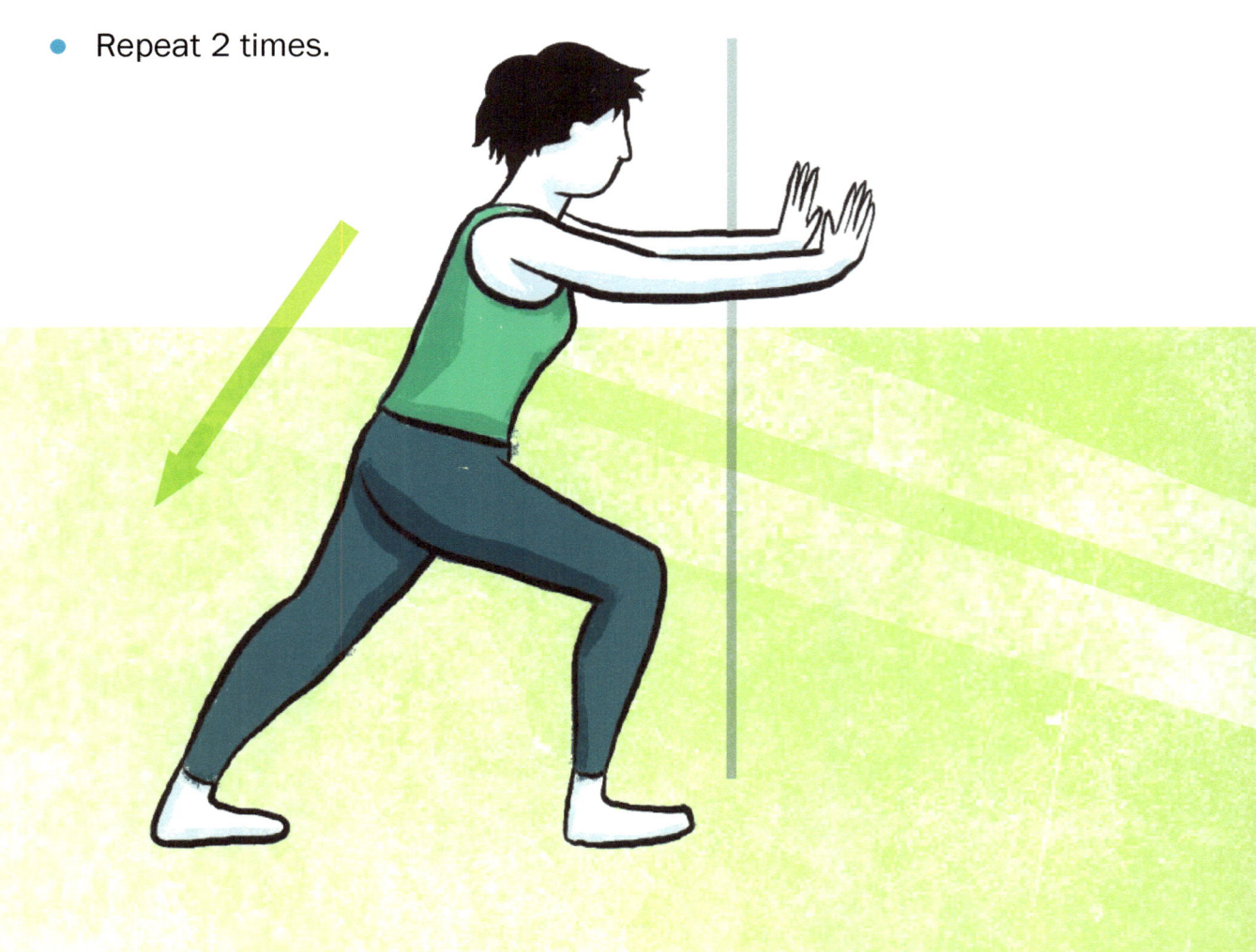

hip stretch

- Sit with legs straight with floor.

- Cross right foot over left leg and place it on the floor. Hold right knee with left arm and pull it in toward your chest as you turn your head and right shoulder toward the right and backwards. Hold 20 to 30 seconds. Return to starting position. Repeat with left foot over your right leg.

- Repeat 2 times.

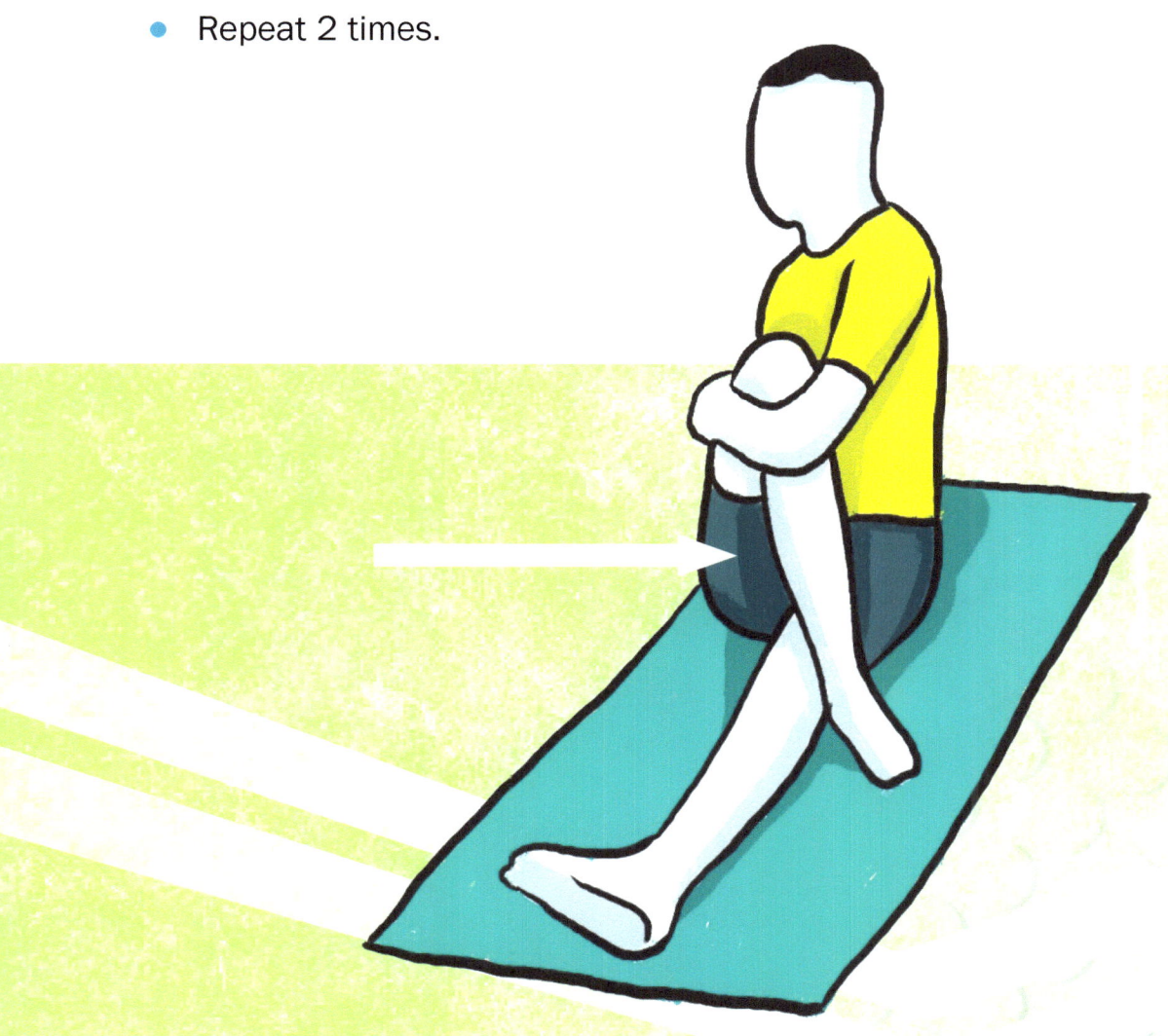

groin stretch

- Sit with bottom of feet together. Hold ankles with hands and push knees gently toward floor with forearms and elbows. Don't force the stretch.

- Sit up tall and lean forward from hips. Hold for 20 to 30 seconds. Return to starting position.

- Repeat 2 times.

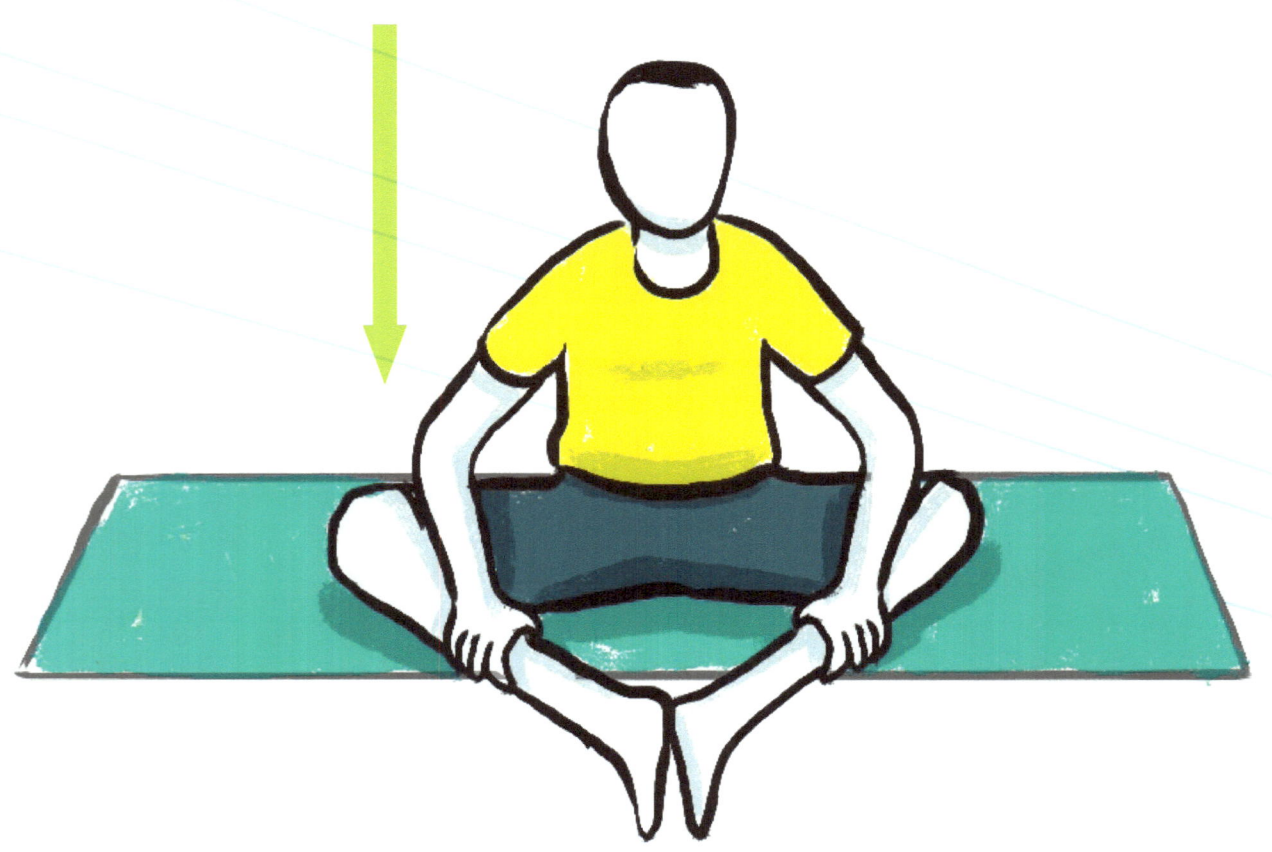

lower back strecth (easier)

- Lie flat on back.

- Bend knees; with both hands, pull thighs toward chest. Hold for 20 to 30 seconds. Return to starting position.

- Repeat 2 times.

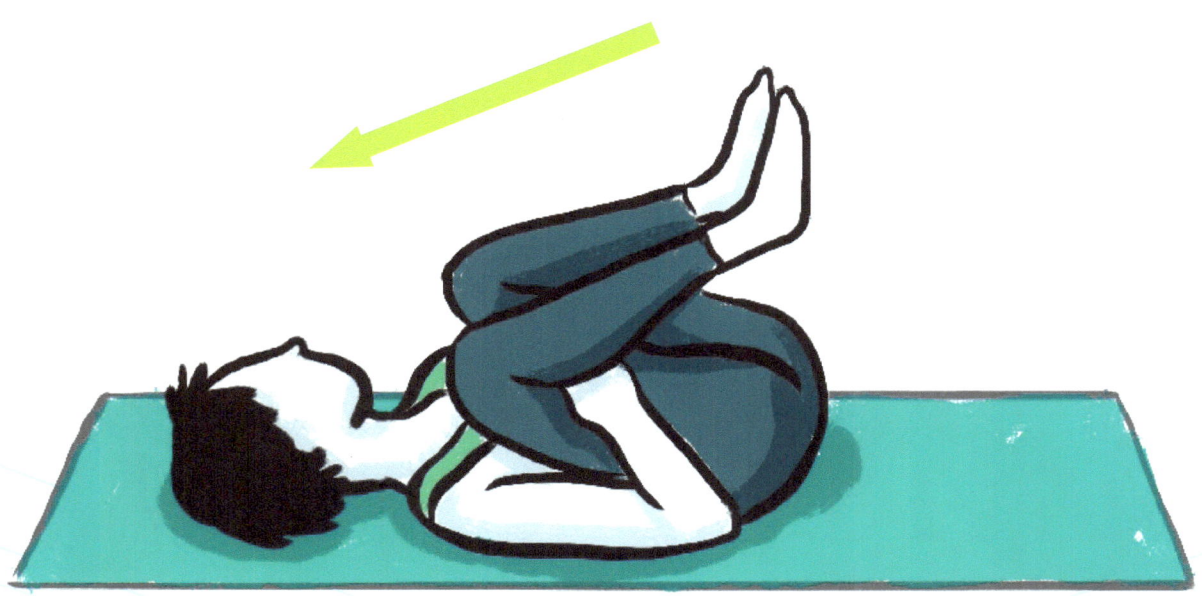

lower back stretch (harder)

- Lie flat on back.

- Bend right knee; pull knee with both hands toward chest. Keep left leg, head and low back flat on floor. Hold 20 to 30 seconds. Return to starting position. Repeat with left leg.

- Repeat 2 times

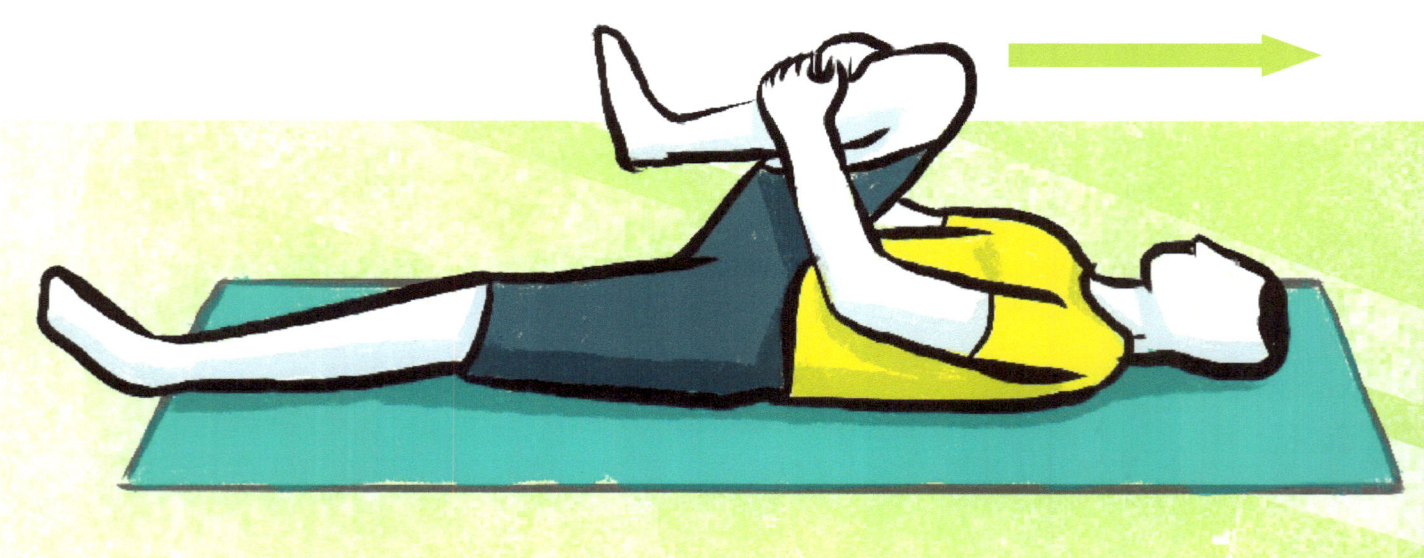

hamstring stretch

- Lie flat on back with right leg bent at knee and right foot flat on floor.

- Keep your left leg straight. Lift left leg straight up. Pull left leg behind your thigh with your hands. Try to point your left toes toward your head. Hold position 20 to 30 seconds. Return left leg to floor. Repeat with left knee bent and lifting right leg.

- Repeat 2 times.

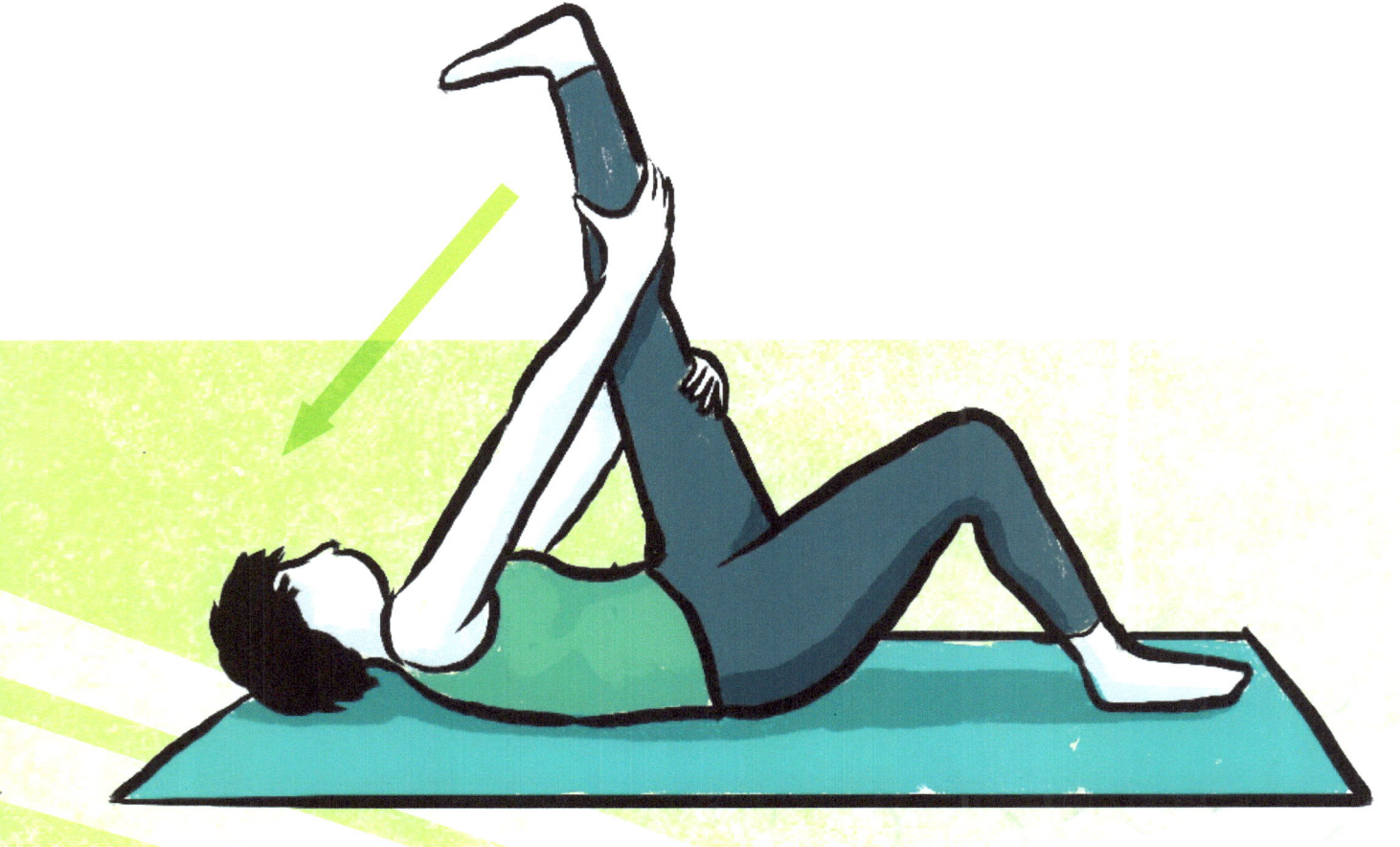

mad cat back stretch

- Put hands and knees on floor. Place hands shoulder width apart.

- Round back upwards. Hold 20 to 30 seconds then slowly relax back to a flat back (do not drop stomach). Tilt your hips and lift your face and chin.

- Repeat 2 times.

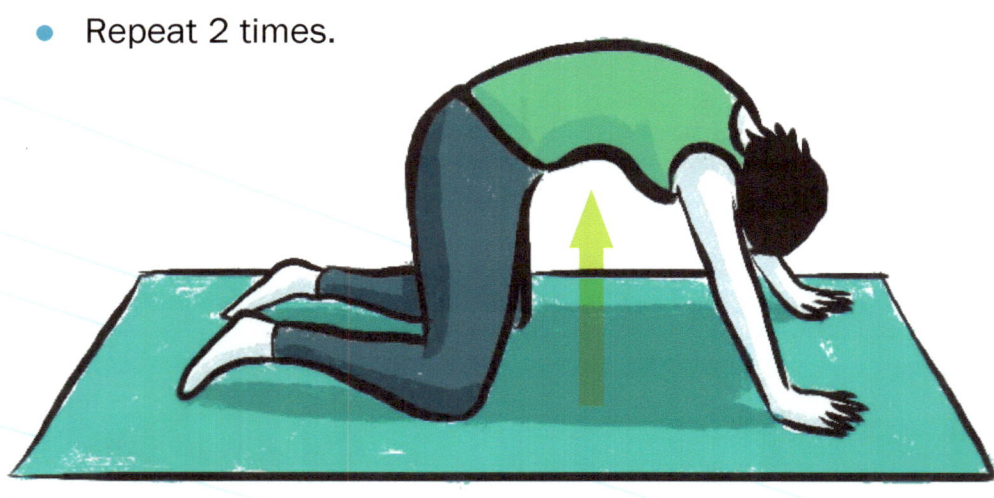

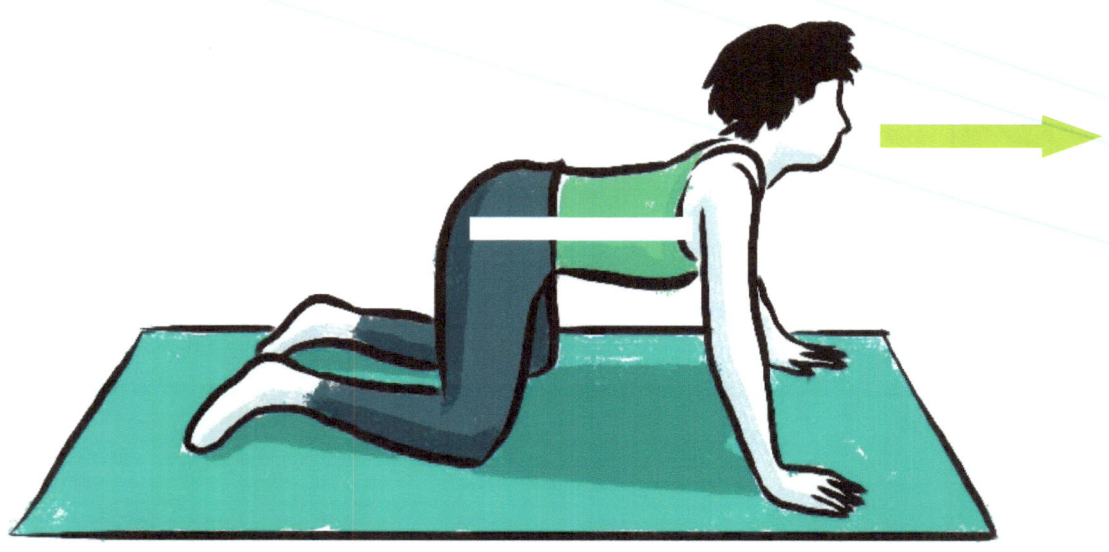

chest/arm/
low-back stretch

- Sit back toward your heels. Lower the upper body toward floor while keeping arms straight.

- Hold 20 to 30 seconds before lifting your upper body to the starting position.

- Repeat 2 times.

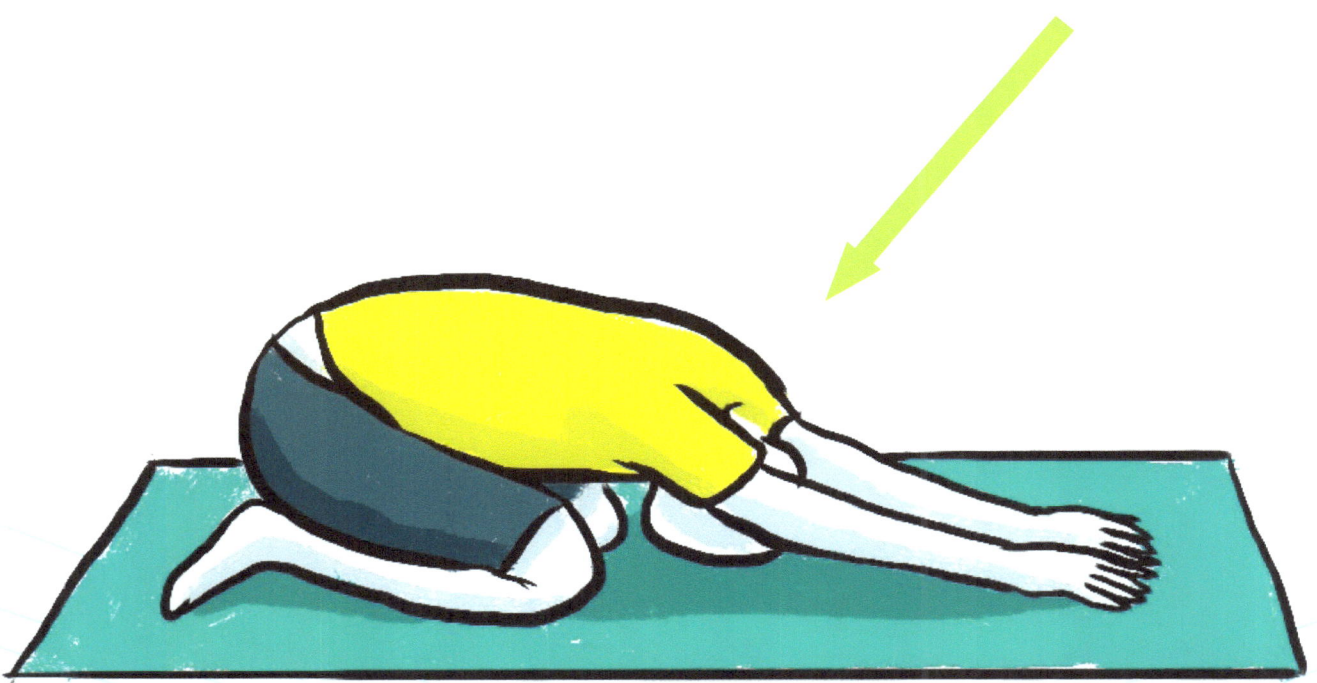

41

supine leg raise

- Lie on your back with right leg bent, foot on the floor, left leg straight.

- Squeeze the muscles on the front of the left thigh and lift the left leg up to knee level of the right leg. Then slowly lower.

- Repeat 10 to 15 times.

- Do the same exercise with right leg 10 to 15 times.

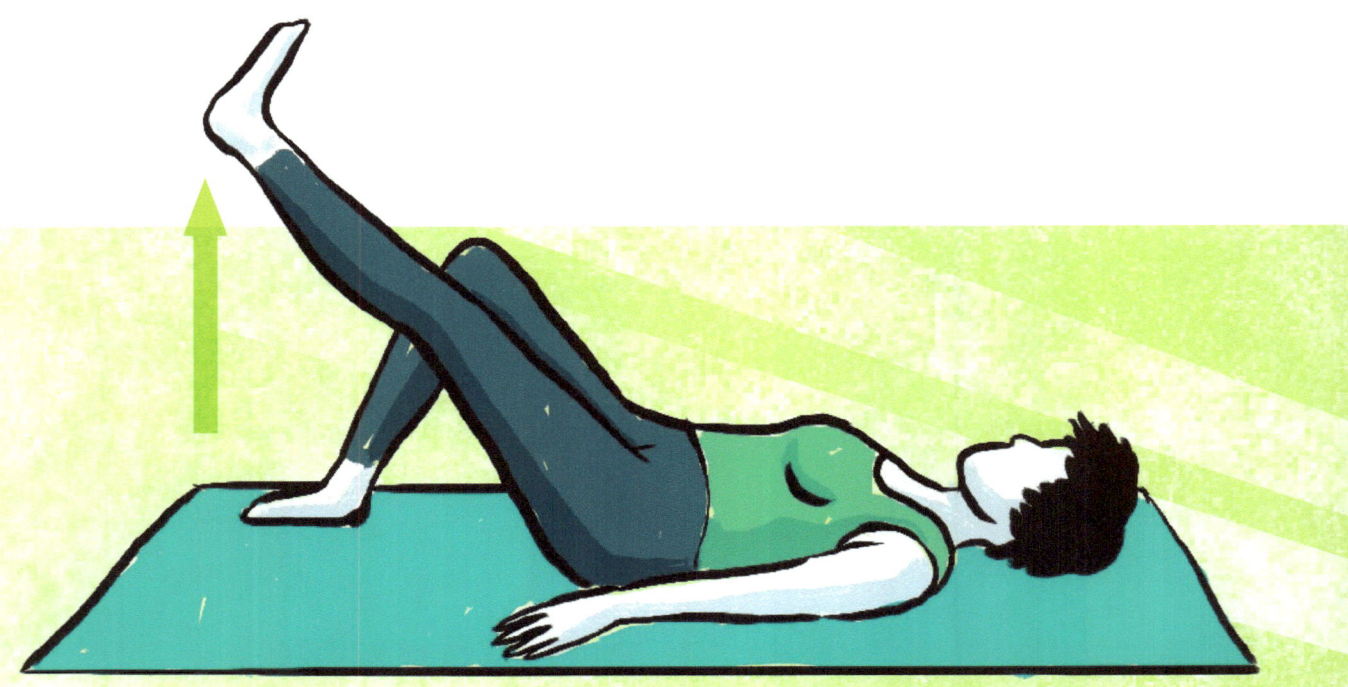

inner thigh leg lift

- Lie on left side with head resting on left arm. Place right foot on floor in front of left leg.

- Keep left leg straight and in line with your body, and lift it off the floor as high as you can. This may be 1 inch to several inches.

- Slowly relax leg to floor.

- Repeat 10 to 15 times.

- Turn over and do the exercise with right leg 10 to 15 times.

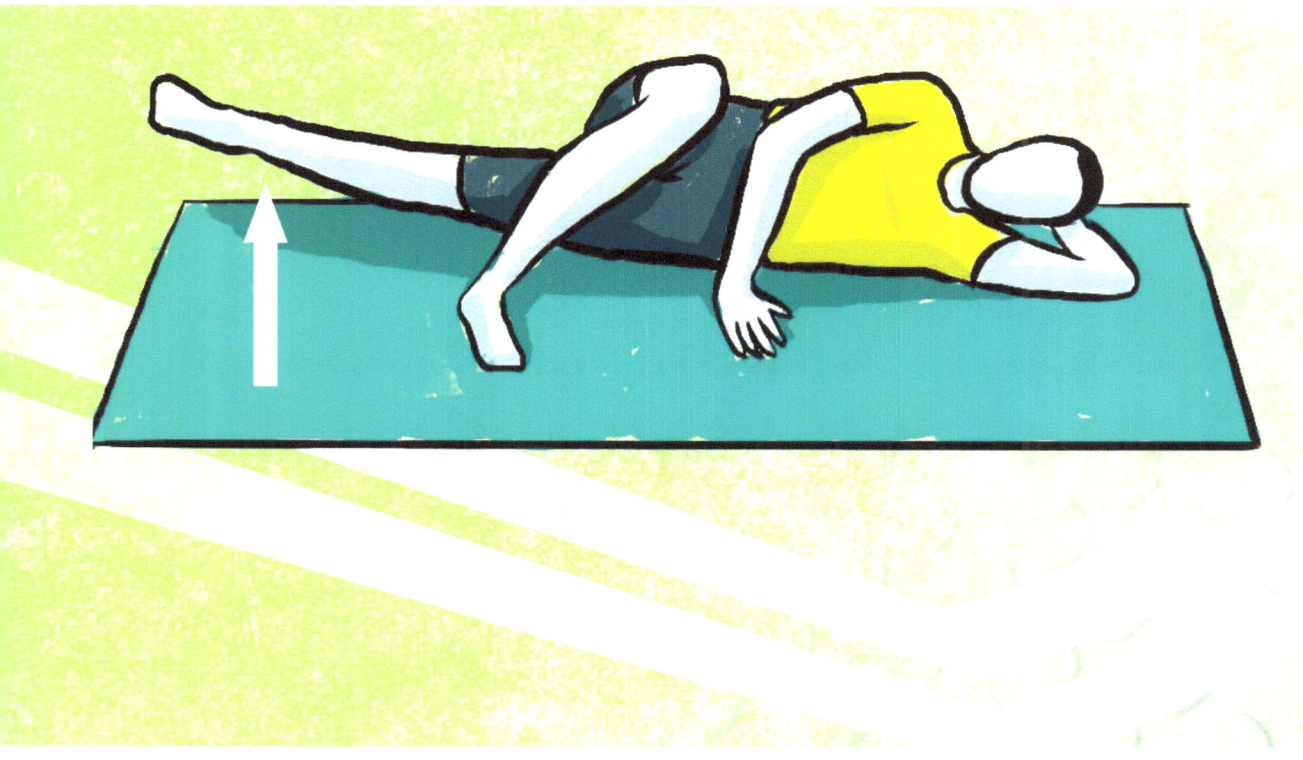

bent knee sit-ups (easier)

- Lie on back with knees bent and feet flat on floor; arms across your chest.

- Squeeze stomach muscles to lift shoulders and head off floor just an inch or two. Keep eyes on ceiling. Slowly lower shoulders back to floor.

- Repeat 10 to 15 times.

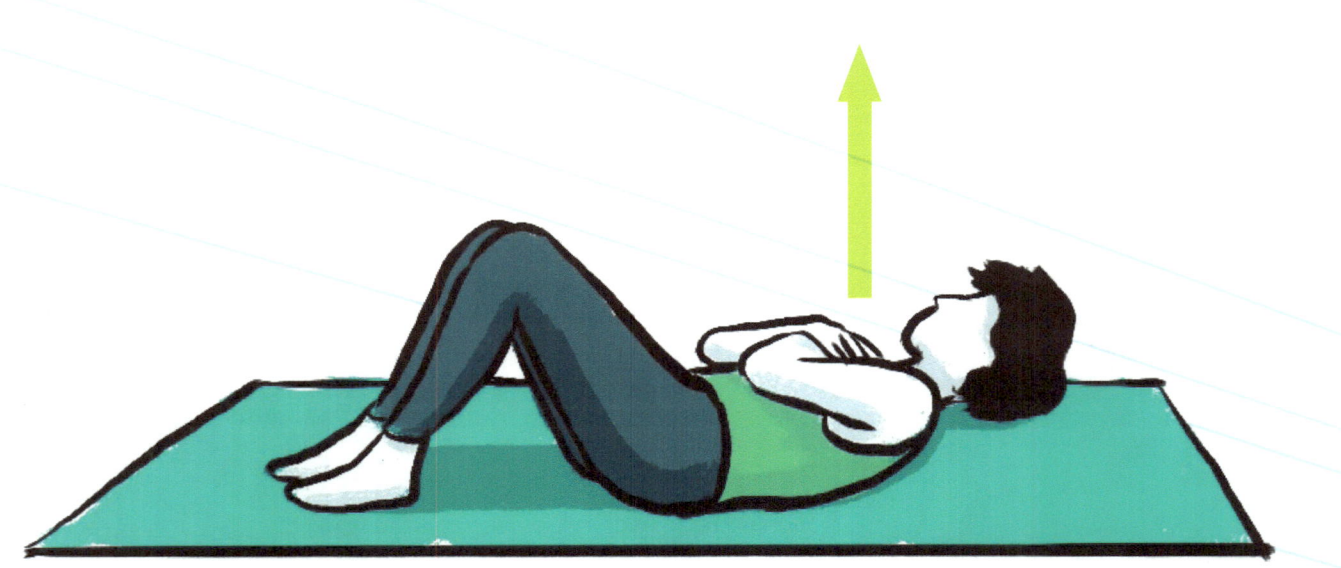

bent knee sit-ups (harder)

- Lie on back with knees bent and feet flat on floor; hands behind your head.

- Squeeze stomach muscles to lift shoulders and head off floor just an inch or two. Keep eyes on ceiling. Slowly lower shoulders back to floor. Don't pull on head or neck.

- Repeat 10 to 15 times.

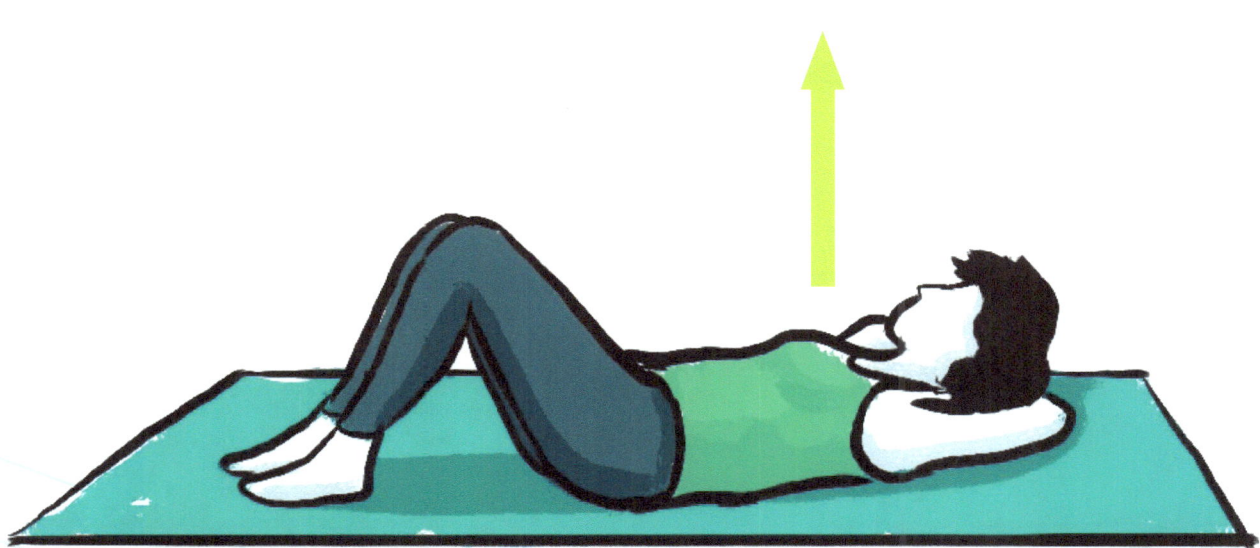

pelvic tilt

- Lie on back with hips and knees bent, feet flat on floor.

- Tighten your stomach muscles and roll your pelvis up and back to flatten your back on the floor.

- Hold for 5 seconds, relax. Repeat 10 to 15 times.

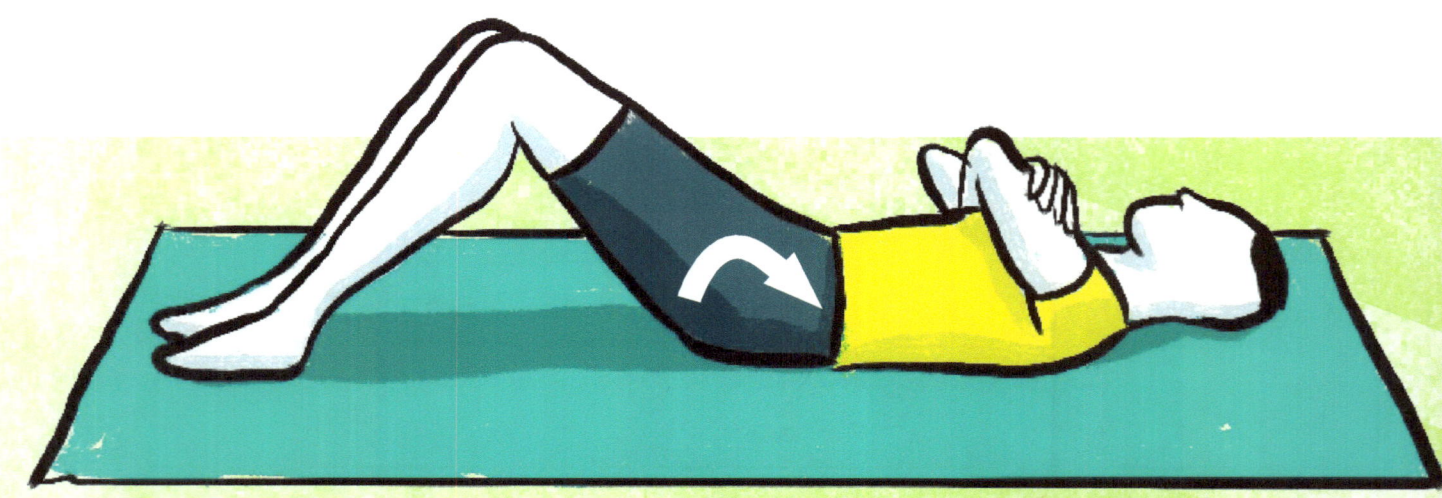

push-ups (easier)

- Lie face down. Put hands under shoulders with palms down. Bend knees with legs together and feet raised slightly off floor.

- Push body (except for hands and knees) off floor. Arms should reach a straight position. Lower body down towards the floor, keeping the body in a straight line from knees to shoulders.

- Repeat 10 to 15 times.

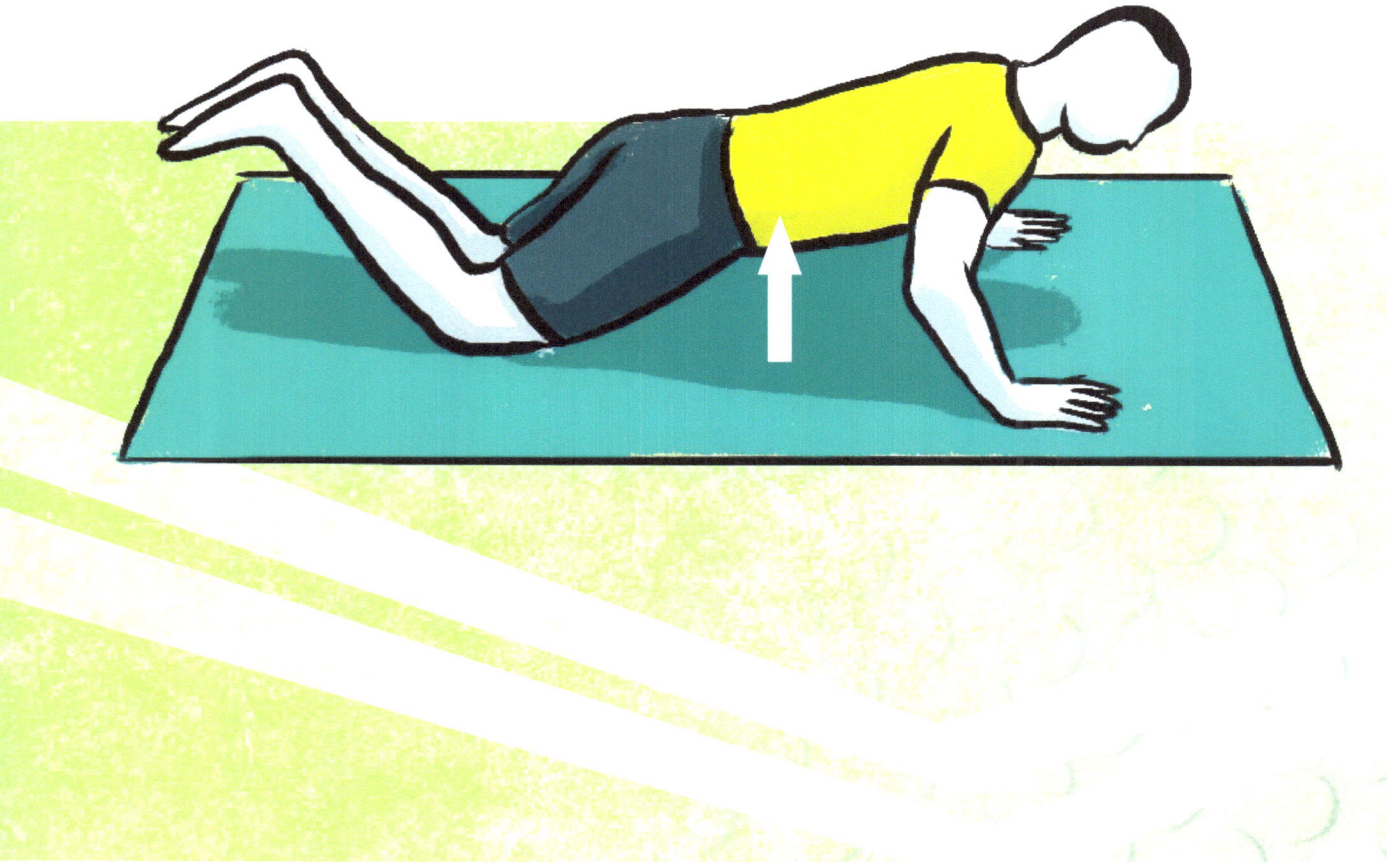

push-ups (harder)

- Lie face down. Put hands under shoulders with palms down. Keep legs together and straight.

- Push body off the floor, keeping back, hips and legs in a straight line.

- Repeat 10 to 15 times.

Try these only if you are able to do 15 of the easier push-ups.

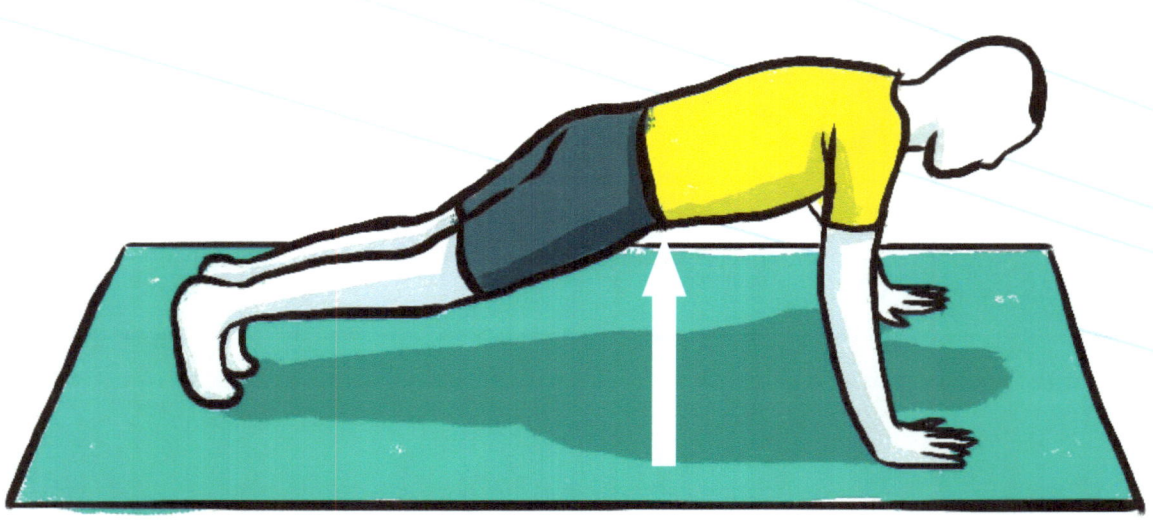

back leg raise

- Put hands and knees on floor. Place hands shoulder width apart.

- Keep back straight, stomach muscles pulled in.

- Extend right leg behind you, knee straight.

- Squeeze buttocks to lift right leg no higher than shoulder level. Do not let back arch. Return to floor.

- Repeat 10 to 15 times with right leg, then 10 to 15 times with left leg.

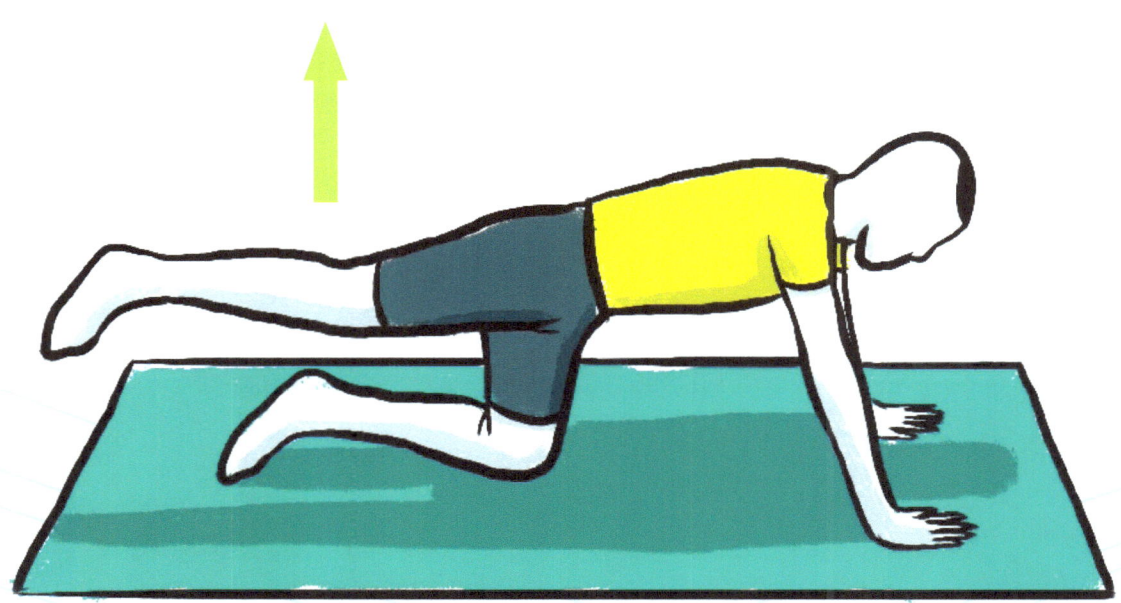

squats (partial)

- Stand tall with feet 18" to 20" apart, toes pointed forward.

- Keeping body erect and heels on floor, slowly bend knees about ¼ to ⅓ of the way down.

- Squeeze hips and thighs to return to starting position.

- Repeat 10 to 15 times.

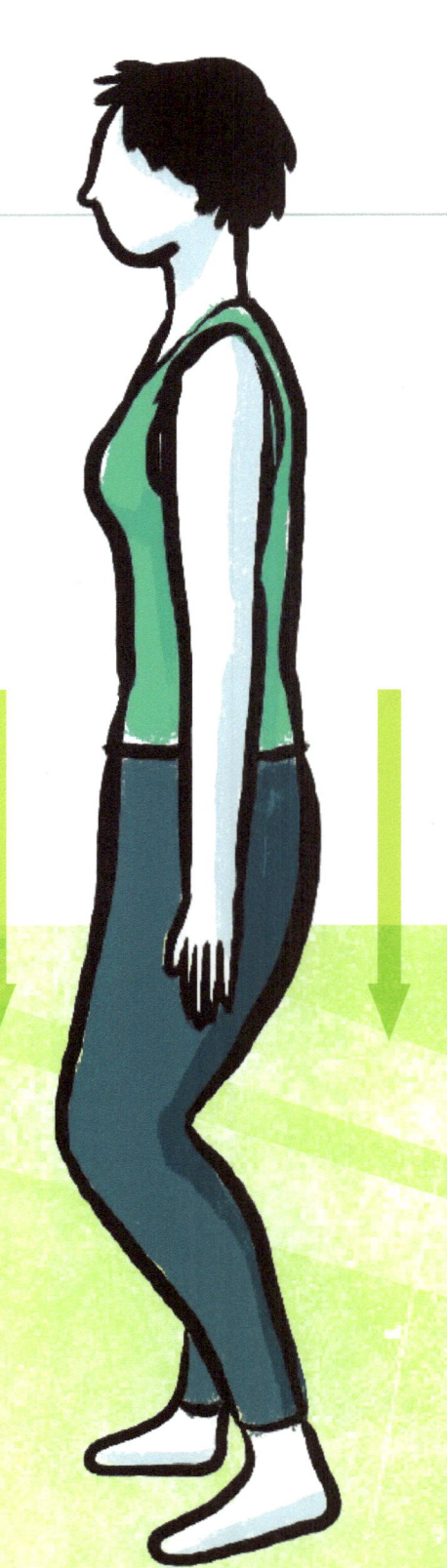

leg raises (standing)

- Stand tall with left hand holding on to a wall or chair for balance. Squeezing hip and stomach muscles, move right leg to right side so that right foot is 8 to 12 inches above floor. Return to starting position.

- Repeat 10 to 15 times.

- Turn around and do exercise with left leg 10 to 15 times.

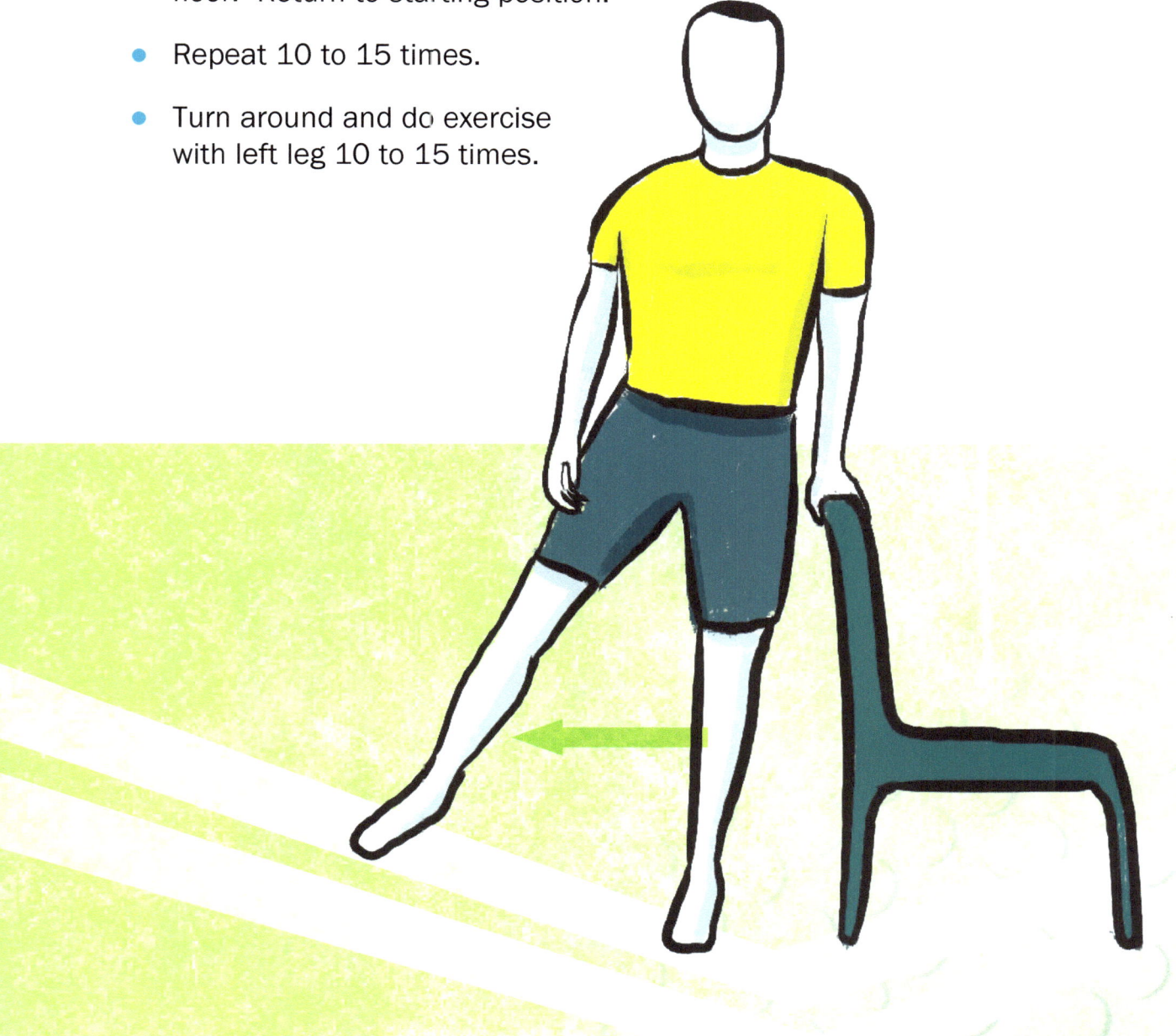

toe-heel lift

- Standing tall, press up onto the balls of the feet.

- Slowly release down. Then curl toes up so you are standing on your heels.

- Repeat 10 to 15 times.

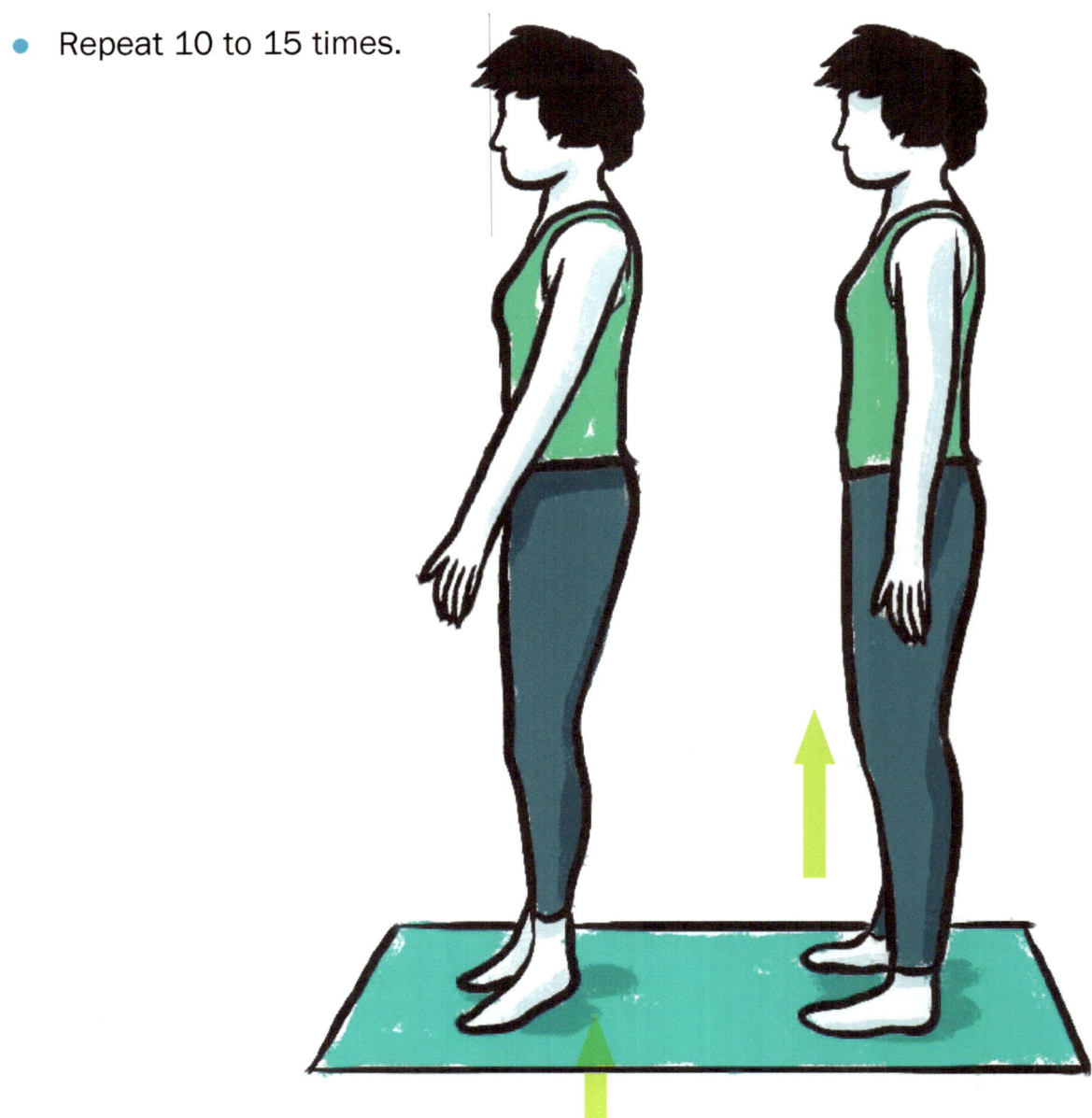

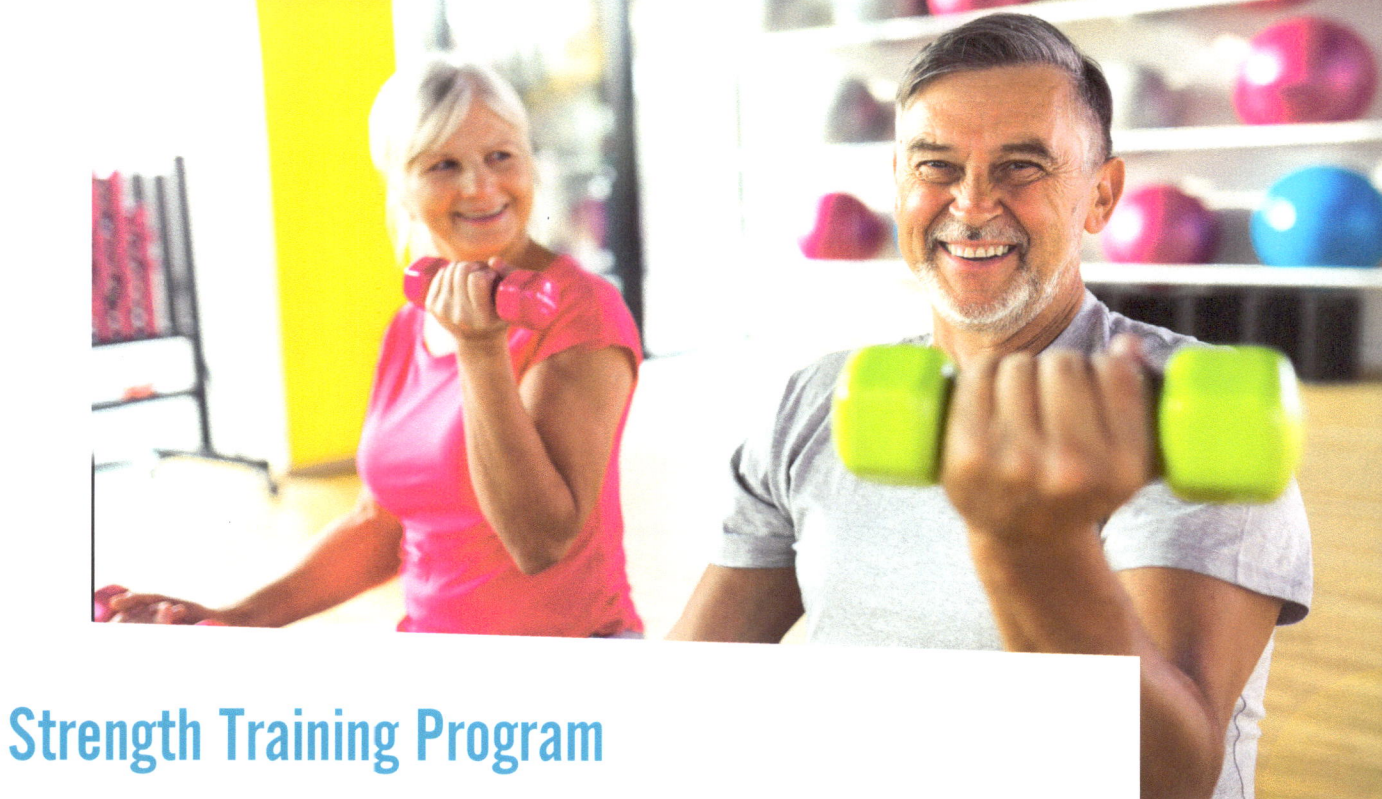

Strength Training Program

1. Lift weights 2 to 3 times a week. Have at least one day between days you weight train. Spend at least 15 minutes in each weight training session.

2. Start with the large muscles—those of the legs and hips. Finish with the smaller muscle groups—chest and arms.

3. Start with light weights (1 to 2 lbs), and see if you can lift them 10 to 15 times. If it is very easy, add more weight. If it is very hard, take some away. You do not have to lift a lot of weight to gain strength. You want to feel resistance, not strain.

4. Use good body posture when lifting weights. Keep your stomach muscles pulled in to help keep your back straight. Never jerk the weights.

5. How and when you breathe is also important with weight training. Breathe deeply the whole time you work with weights. Breathe out as you lift the weight, and breathe in as you lower the weight.

6. If you have had open heart surgery, check with your HCP first to find out which strength building exercises are right for you.

squat

Muscles used: Front and back of thighs, hips

Body position: Hold weight in each hand at side of body. Place feet 18 to 20 inches apart, toes pointed forward.

Movement: Keeping body erect as you can, bend knees and lower body only ¼ to ⅓ of the way down. Do not let heels come off of the floor. Squeeze hips and back of thighs. Return to start position.

Repeat 10 to 15 times.

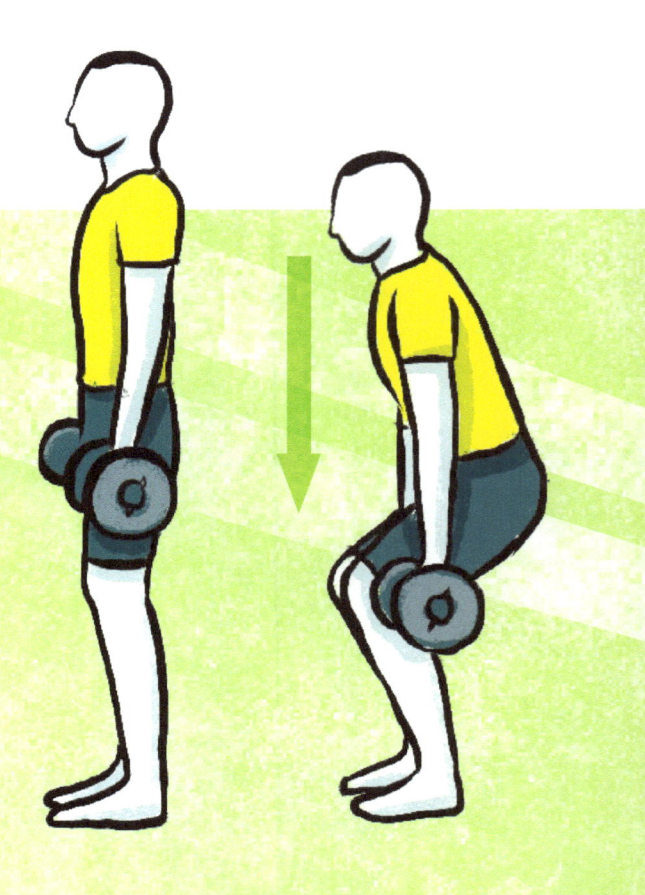

seated calf raise

Muscles used: Back of lower leg

Body position: Sit with two dumbbells supported on thighs and
with ball of each foot up on a thick book or 2 to
3 inch board.

Movement: Squeezing just the calf muscles, press your heels up
as high as you can. Then slowly lower back to floor.

Repeat 10 to 15 times.

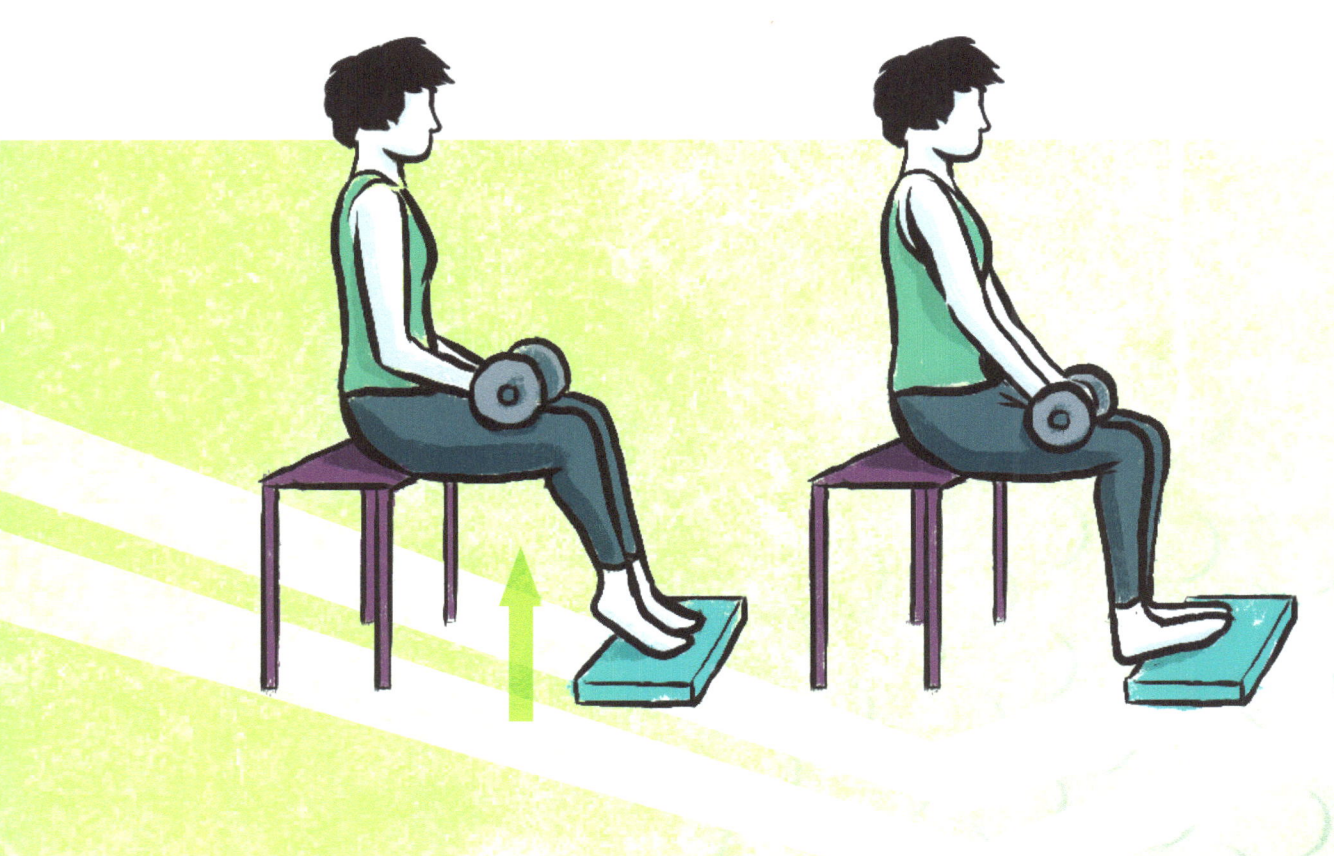

lunge

Muscles used: Front and back of thighs, butt

Body position: Stand with feet hip-width apart, hold weight in each hand, palms facing in.

Movement: Step forward with your right leg and bend the right knee until your upper leg is about level with the floor (90° angle). Keep your weight on your right leg and your spine straight. Push back up on your right leg to your start position. Then do this with your left leg.

Repeat 10 to 15 times.

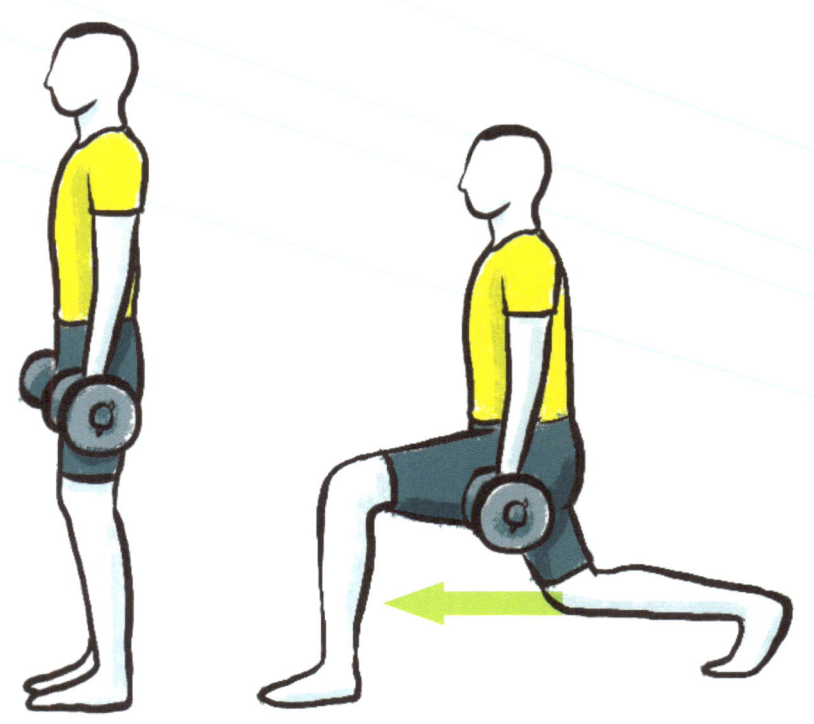

bench press

Muscles used: Chest, front of shoulders, back of arms

Body position: Lie on weight bench with knees bent, feet on end of bench. Hold weight in each hand at chest level.

Movement: Press upward from shoulders. Then slowly lower to start position.

Repeat 10 to 15 times.

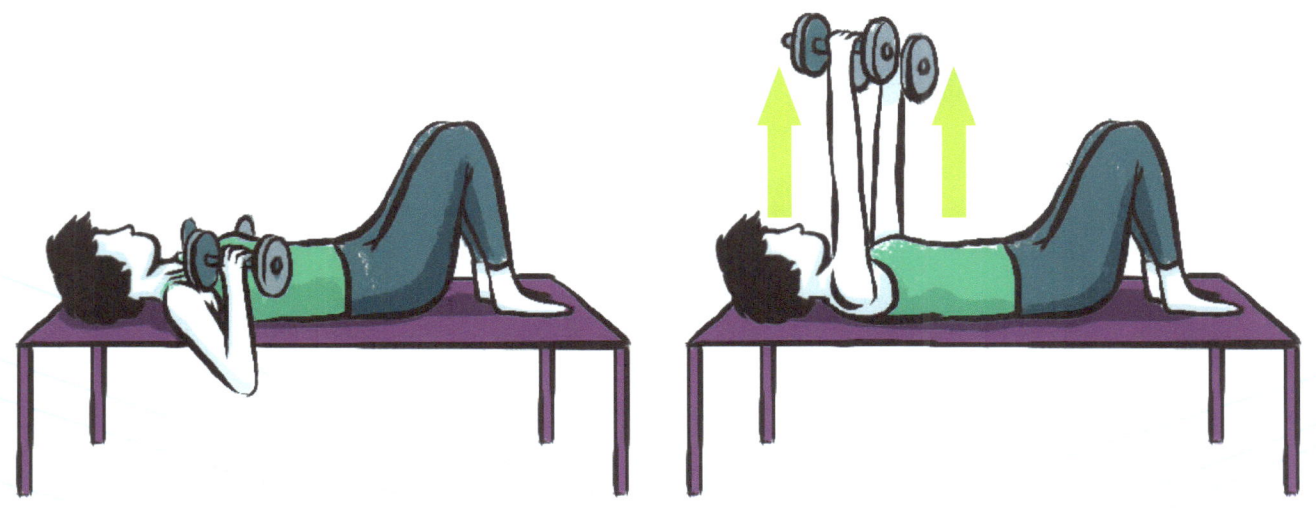

flys

Muscles used: Chest, arms

Body position: Lie on weight bench with knees bent, feet on the
end of bench. Hold weights above chest, arms
nearly straight.

Movement: With elbows slightly bent, slowly lower the weights to
each side until arms are parallel to floor. Return arms
to start position.

Repeat 10 to 15 times.

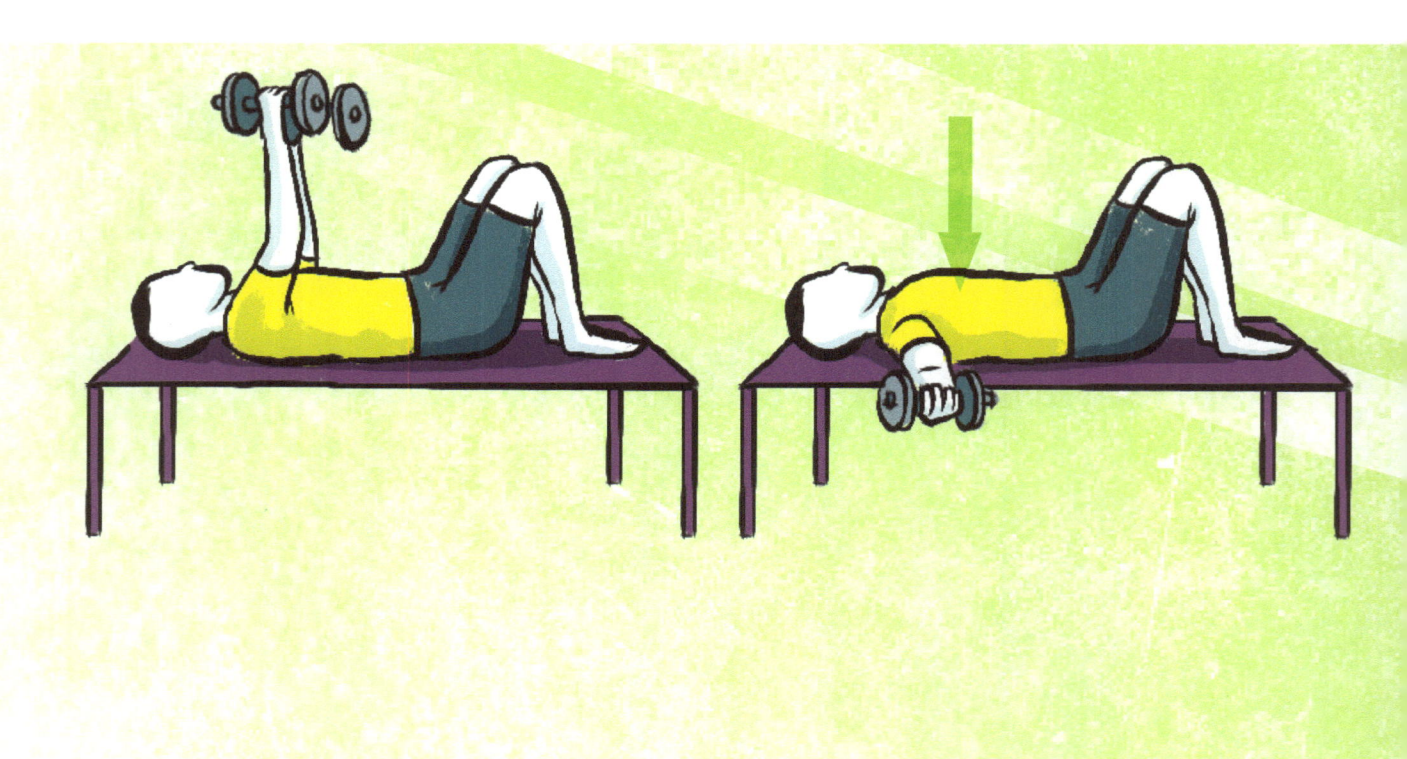

front raise

Muscles used: Shoulders, upper arms

Body position: Stand with feet a little over shoulder-width apart, grasp weights in each hand out in front of you, palms facing your body.

Movement: Look straight ahead and use your shoulder muscles to slowly lift dumbbells out in front of you. Lift until weights are about even with your shoulders. Hold weights and count to 3, then slowly lower weights back to start.

Repeat 10 to 15 times.

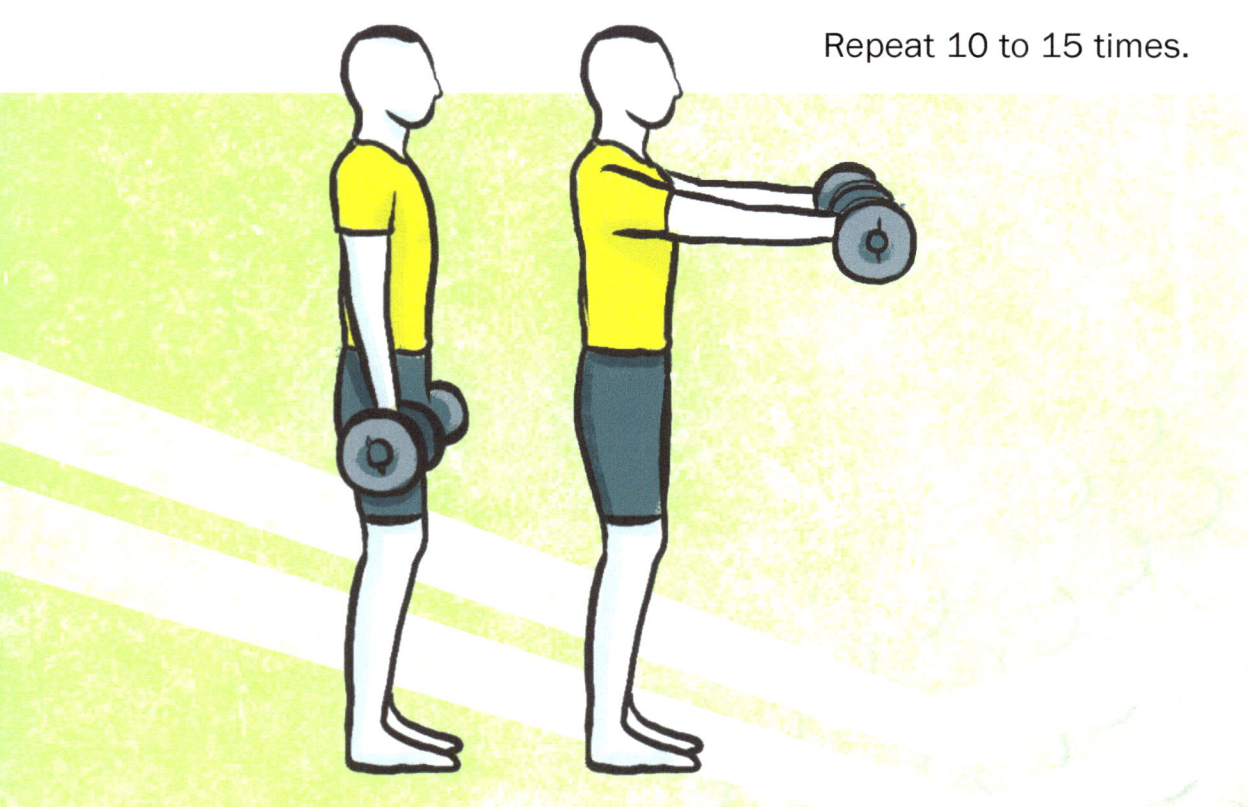

side raise

Muscles used:	Shoulders, upper arms
Body position:	Stand with feet shoulder-width apart, hands at your side. Hold weight in each hand, palms facing in. Hold your shoulders back and chest out, lean slightly forward.
Movement:	Use your shoulder muscles to slowly raise dumbbells out from your side. Lift until weights are parallel with the floor. Hold weights and count to 3, then slowly lower weights back to start.

Repeat 10 to 15 times.

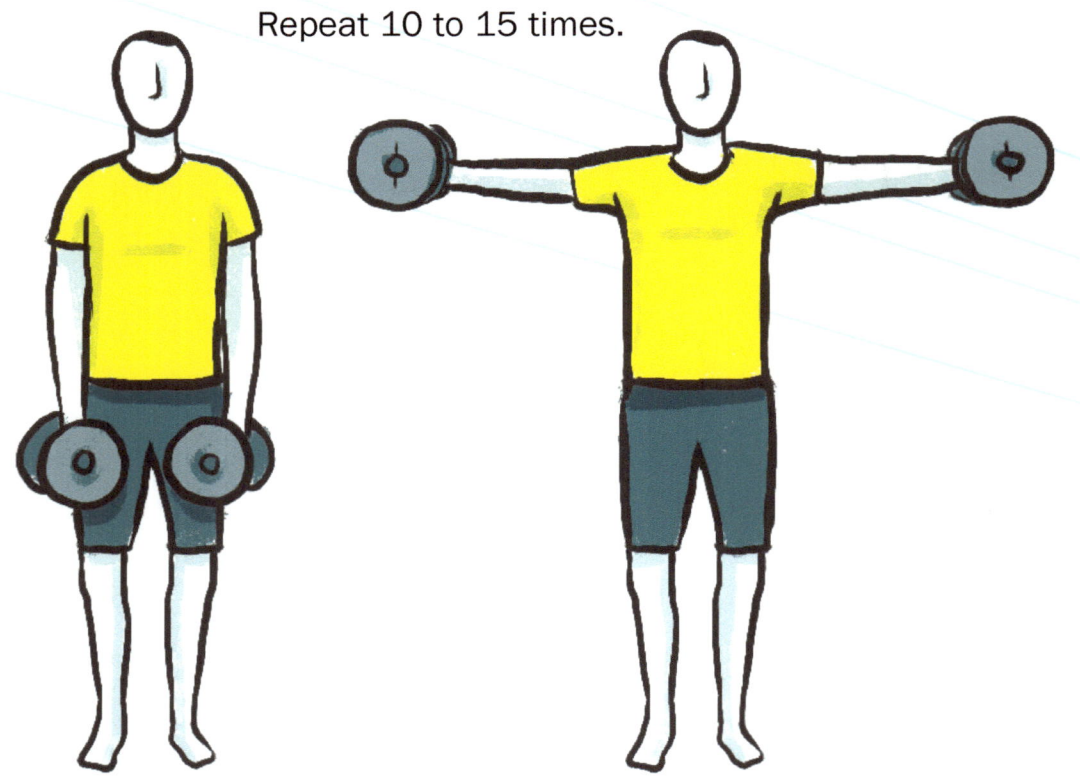

overhead raise

Muscles used: Shoulders, upper arms

Body position: Stand with feet shoulder-width apart, hands at your side. Hold weight in each hand, palms facing in.

Movement: Slowly raise dumbbells up in front of you. Lift until weights are over your head with arms bent. Hold position and count to 3, then slowly lower weights back to start.

Repeat 10 to 15 times.

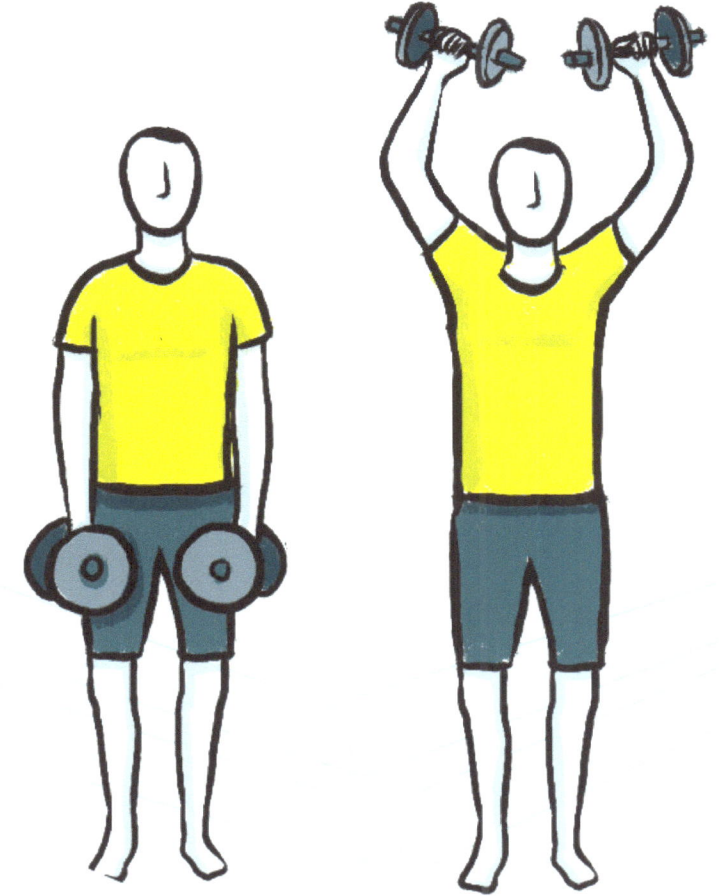

tricep kickback

Muscles used: Shoulders, upper arms

Body position: Stand beside bench, put right knee on bench, bend over and prop up with right hand on bench. Keep left leg out from bench beyond your left shoulder. Grasp dumbbell in left hand, palm side in.

Movement: Slowly pull dumbbell up toward left side of chest. Bring left elbow up as far as you can. Then slowly lower weights back to start. Do not relax muscles and repeat exercise.

Repeat 10 to 15 times. Then reposition with left knee on bench and follow same procedure.

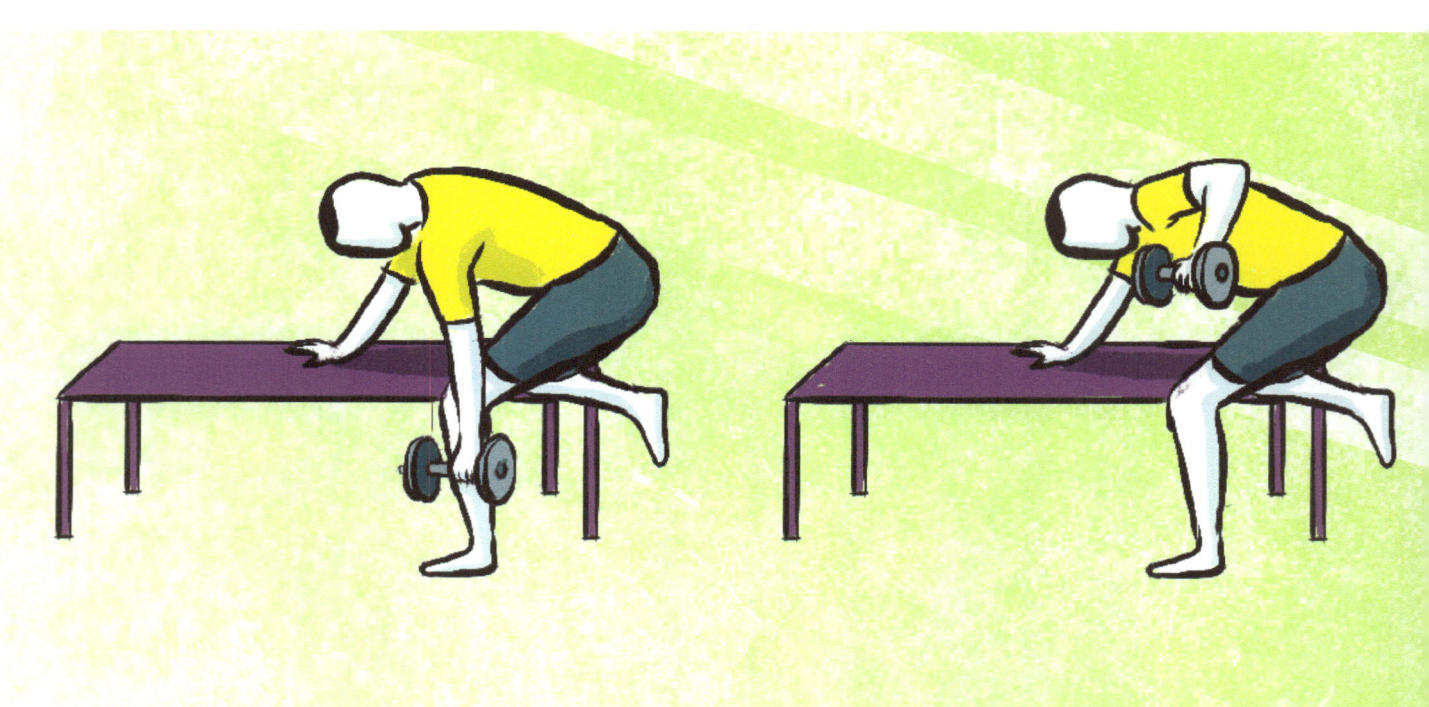

shoulder press

Muscles used: Shoulders, back of arms

Body position: Stand erect, stomach pulled in. Hold weight in each
hand at shoulder level.

Movement: Raise weights above the head without letting your
back arch. Slowly return to start position.

Repeat 10 to 15 times.

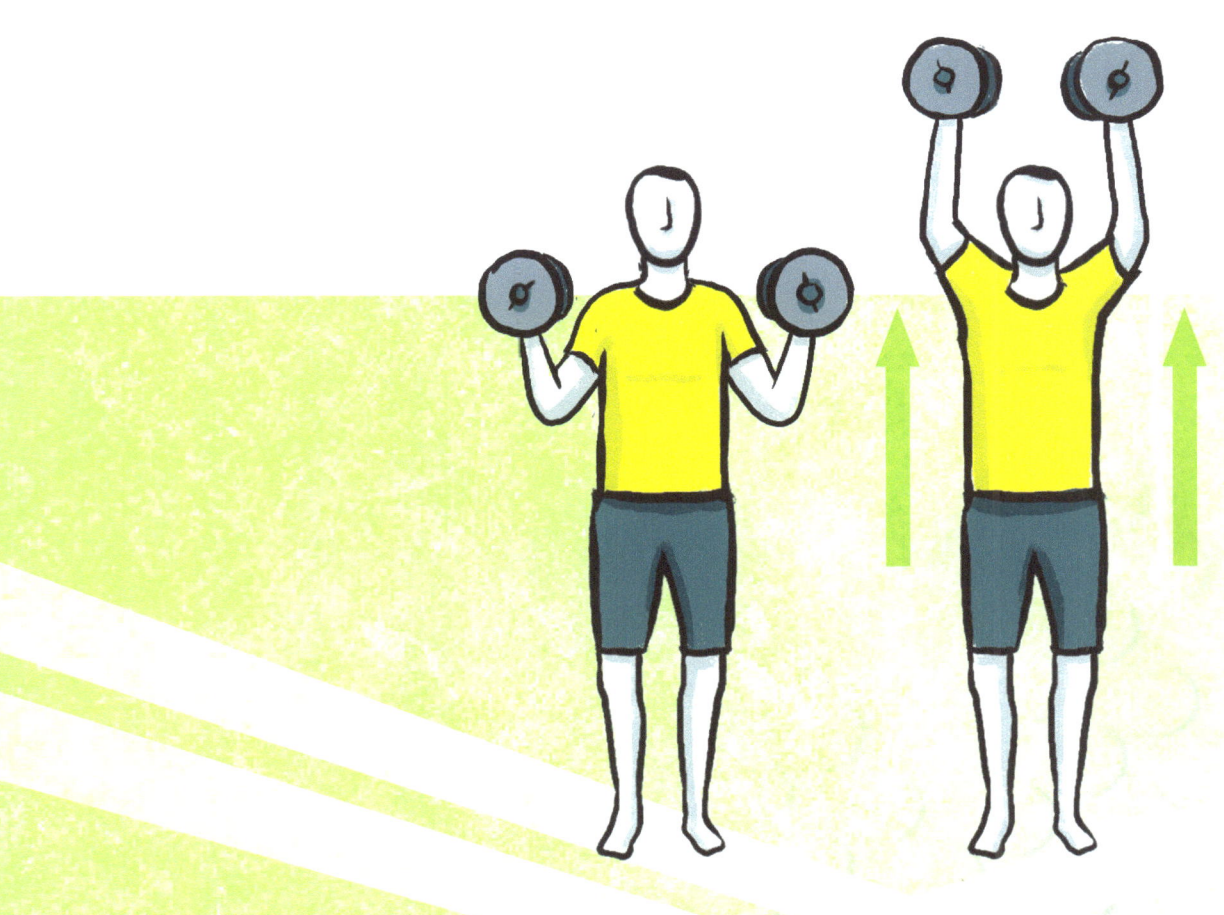

side bends

Muscles used: Back, shoulders

Body position: Stand with feet shoulder-width apart. Hold dumbbell at your side with your right hand, palm side in. Knees slightly bent.

Movement: Slowly bend your body to the right, without bending forward, as far as you comfortably can, letting weight hang out from side. Hold while you count to 3. Return to start and repeat 10 to 15 times.

Then hold dumbell at your left side, palm in and repeat as above.

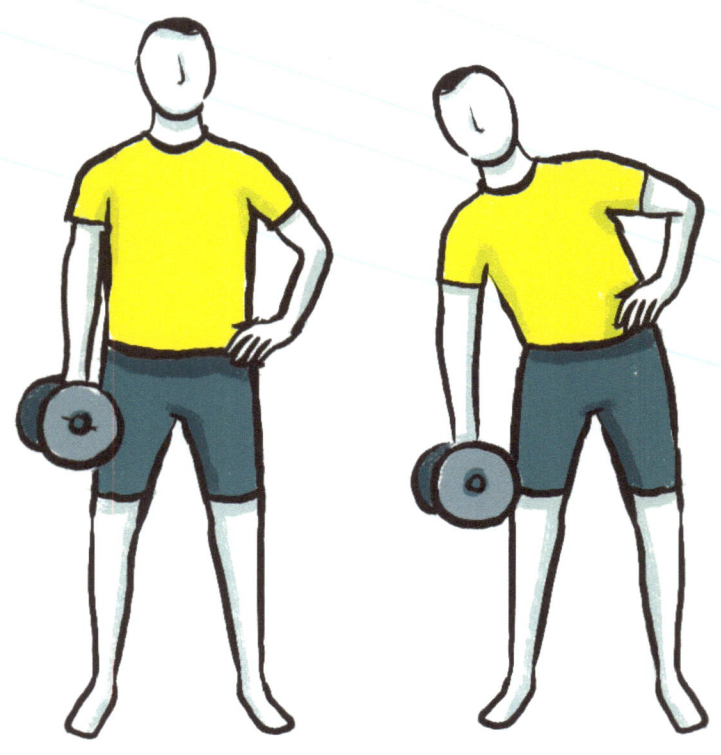

tricep extension

Muscles used: Back of upper arms

Body position: Grab dumbbells with palms facing in. Lie face up on bench, feet on floor. Hold weights out from body so that upper arms are pointed toward the ceiling.

Movement: Bend elbows to bring weights down beside head.

Repeat 10 to 15 times.

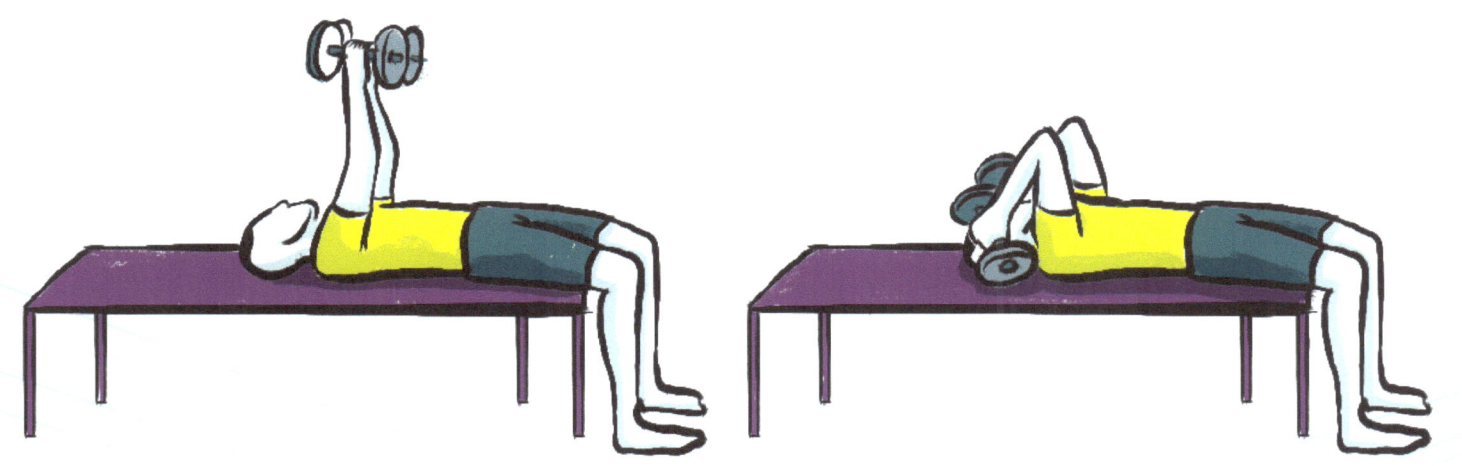

arm curls

Muscles used: Upper and lower arm muscles

Body position: Stand with feet 18 to 24 inches apart. Hold weights with palms up. Keep arms and back straight.

Movement: Bend elbows and curl your arms up until the weight nearly touches your chest. Do not jerk the weight.

Repeat 10 to 15 times.

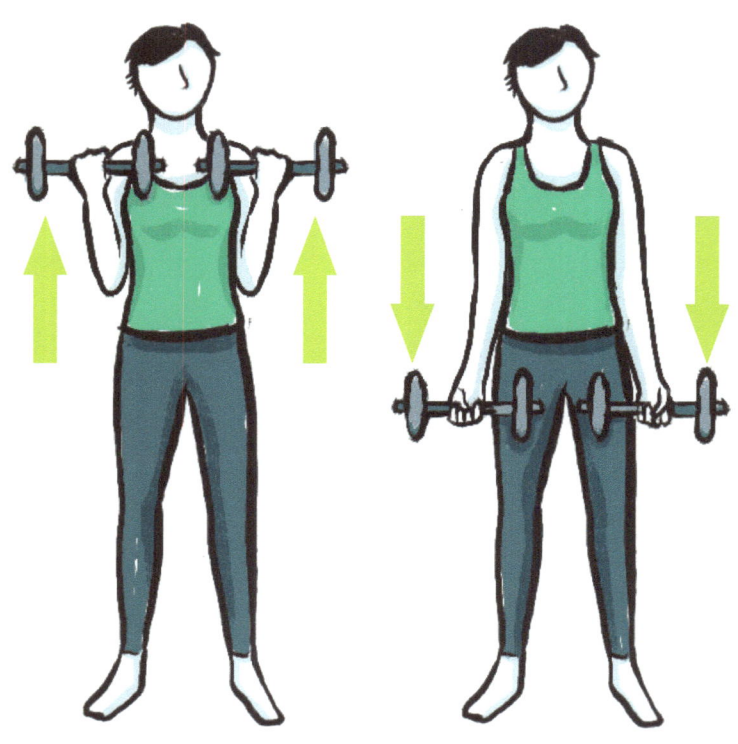

Environment

Exercise can be done almost anywhere. Yet the world outdoors can give you problems. Knowing what to do about the weather and knowing how to dress will add to your safety and fun.

heat, humidity, fluids

Body temperature is balanced by the heat the body produces and the heat it loses. This keeps the body temperature at 98.6° (37°C). When body temperature goes up, blood vessels become larger, and blood moves to the skin's surface. As you sweat, heat leaves the body, and the skin and blood are cooled. The cooled blood then carries oxygen back to the working muscles.

In hot and/or humid weather, you have to help your body stay cool. You may also need to do this when you exercise for a long time. In hot weather, your body must not only deal with its own heat but also the hot air around it. The loss of body heat by sweating may not be enough to cool the skin and blood. If this happens, be sure to:

- **drink water**– about one cup every 20 minutes of exercise

- **wet your skin with water,** especially if you do not sweat

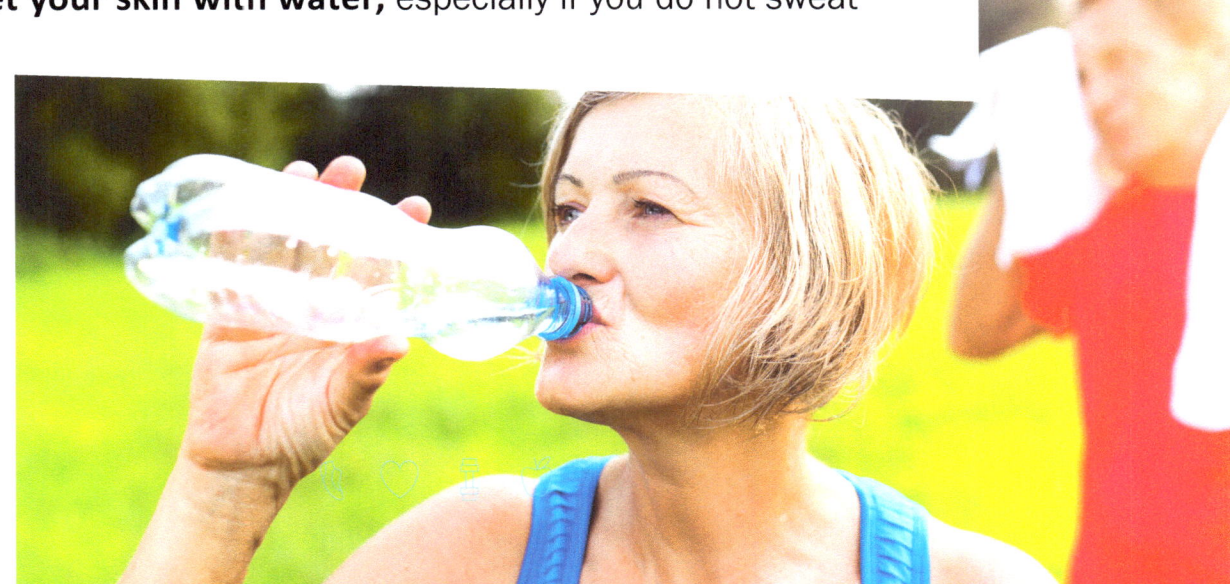

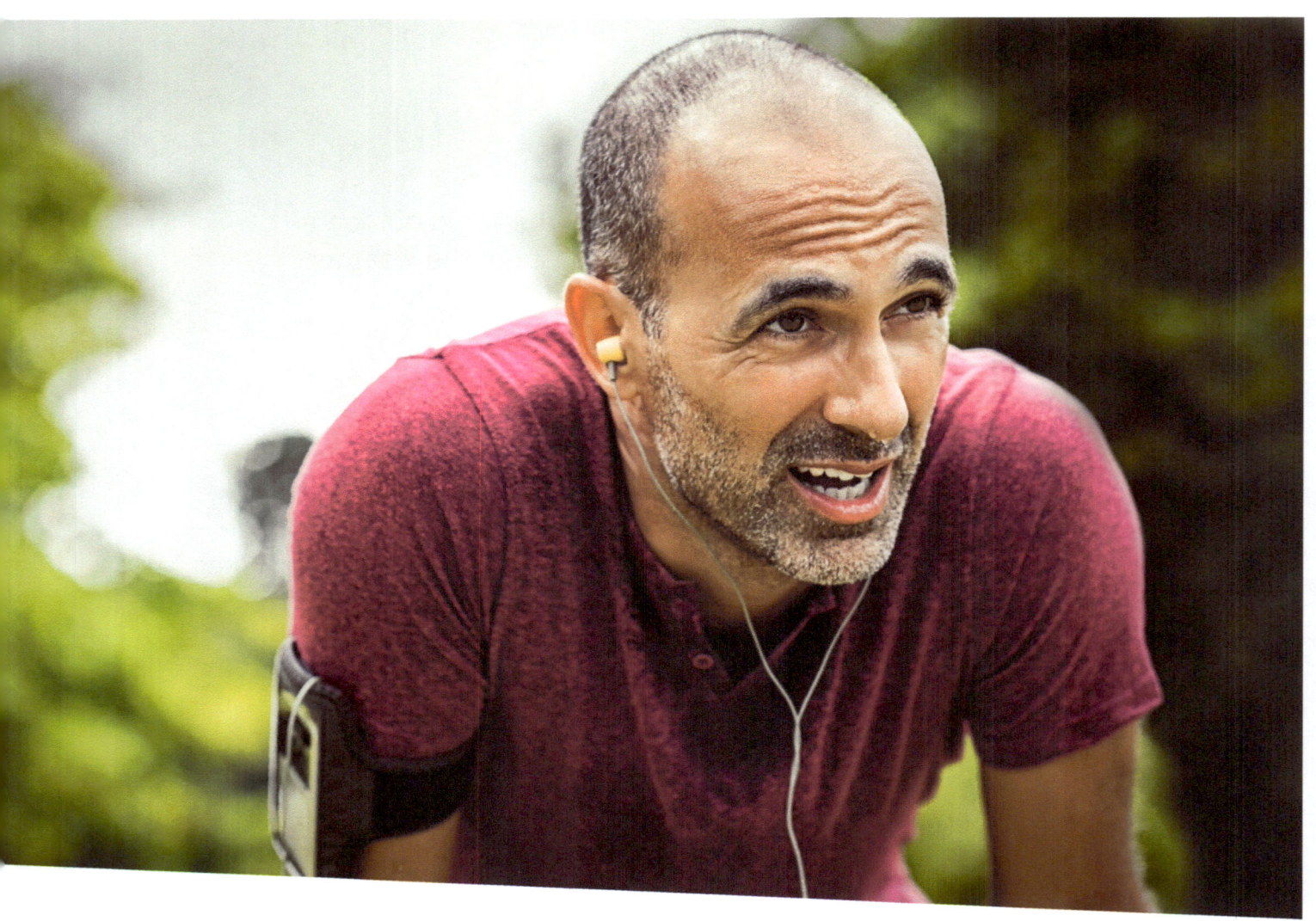

You must replace fluids and keep the body cool to avoid heat sickness or dehydration. Hot weather does not bother physically trained people as much as it does beginners. **Beginners should limit exercise time** in very hot weather. But even people who exercise at high levels need to drink fluids and know when to stop before getting too hot.

If you have a heart problem and the weather is hot (above 95°) and humid (80% or more), reduce the time you exercise outdoors by 25%. Exercise indoors is fine if the room is properly cooled.

cold weather

While hot weather expands blood vessels, cold weather narrows them. As blood vessels get smaller, the heart must pump harder to move the same amount of blood through smaller vessels. This can raise blood pressure. Cold weather may also reduce how much air the lungs can exchange. As the body becomes colder, less oxygen is sent to the working muscles. This may or may not be noticed by a healthy, trained person, but **people with heart disease** may feel chest pressure (angina) or have irregular heartbeats. **People with lung disease** may feel more short of breath and not be able to exercise outdoors in very cold weather. It is best to exercise indoors if the outside temperature is 39°F (4°C) or less.

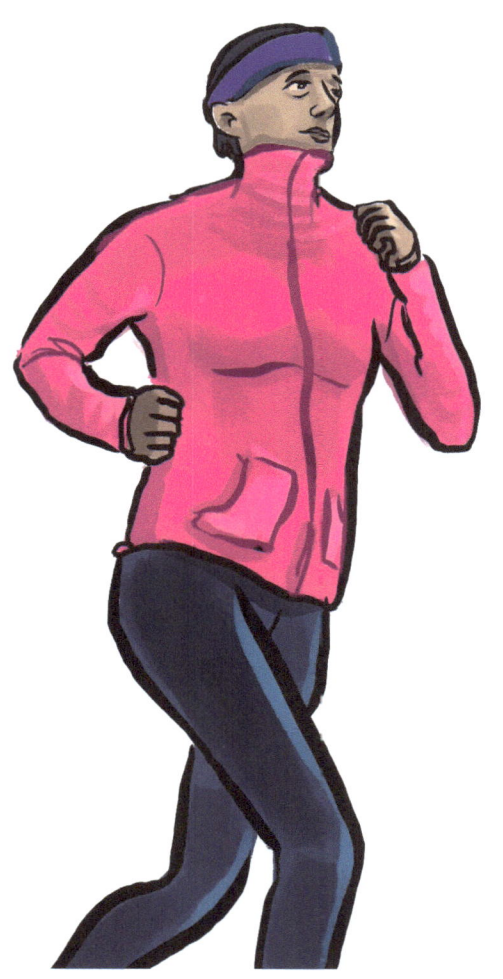

wind

When you exercise against the wind, you may want to slow down or exercise for a shorter time than is normal for you. Wind makes you work harder and makes the body feel colder than it may actually be.

altitude

Healthy people can exercise in altitudes higher than 10,000 feet. You should take a few days to get used to the altitude. But this does not mean that high altitudes will not make a person feel sick. You may still feel sleepy, very tired, sick to your stomach, light-headed or have a headache. These are the signs of altitude sickness. If you feel any of these, do not exercise for a day or two, or descend to a lower altitude. Medicines like Diamox can help prevent symptoms at high altitudes.

People with heart problems can also exercise in high altitudes, but it should be done with care. Many take part in mild activities at altitudes of 6,000 to 8,000 feet. In fact, some ski or vacation in cities located at just under 10,000 feet and enjoy it. But if you have heart problems, do not exercise when you feel sick from the altitude.

surfaces

If you have weak ankles or back or muscle problems, uneven surfaces may give you trouble. Flexibility exercises can help you overcome your body's weak areas. Do them each time you exercise.

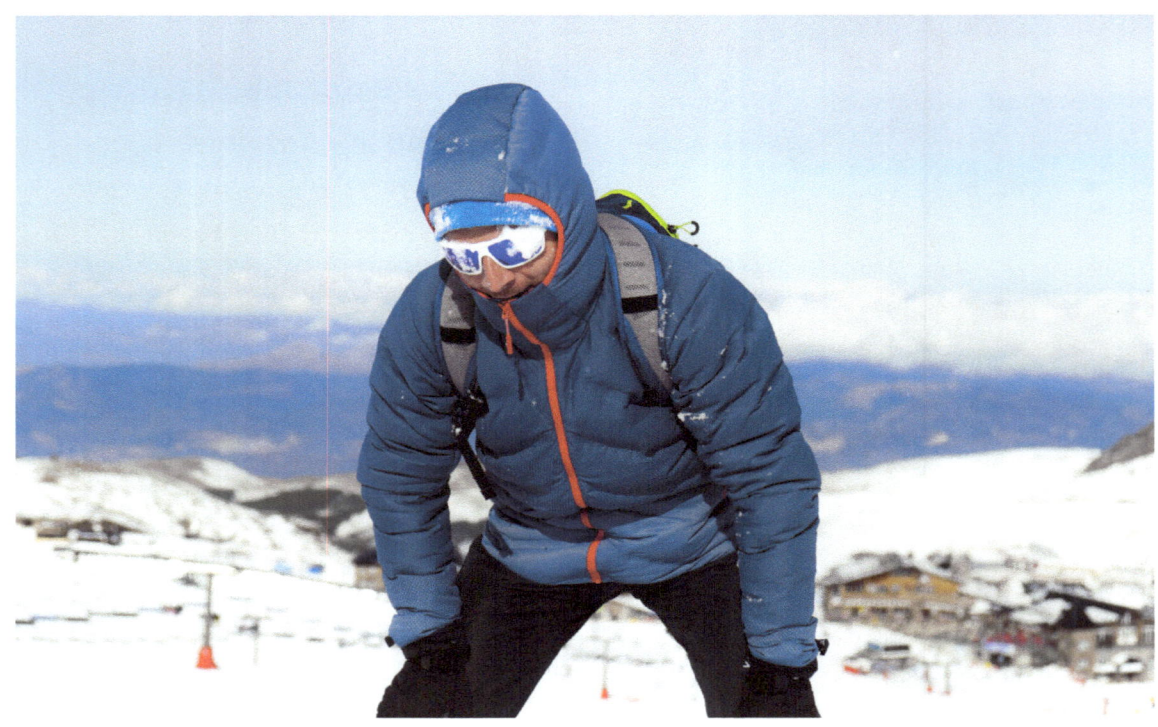

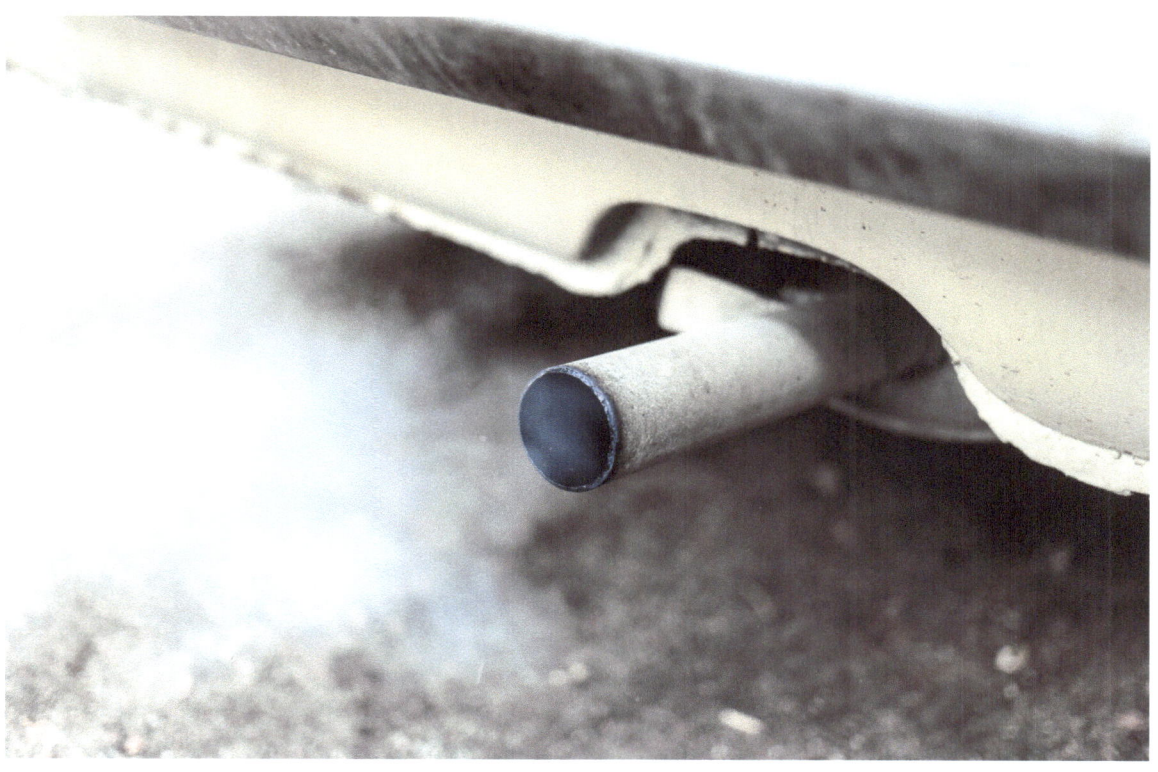

air pollution

It is hard for the body to get oxygen in dirty air. This can be true in air filled with tobacco smoke, industrial fumes, car exhaust and smog. When the body is getting less oxygen, the heart beats faster trying to meet the body's need for more oxygen. This is most true for people with heart or lung disease. So when you know that the air is polluted, **do not do hard exercises.**

Car exhaust is a very common air pollutant. When it is breathed, carbon monoxide replaces some of the oxygen and gets into the blood and goes to the muscles. This can give chest pressure (angina) to people with heart disease. It can also cause irregular heartbeats. Patients with lung disease may feel short of breath.

The normal level of carbon monoxide in the blood is less than 1%. People living in cities with lots of smog may have up to 3% carbon monoxide. So the more pollution in the air, the less oxygen in the blood. Also, remember that smokers have levels of 4 to 10% carbon monoxide.

Smoke-free work places and restaurants have helped reduce the risk from pollutants and smoke.

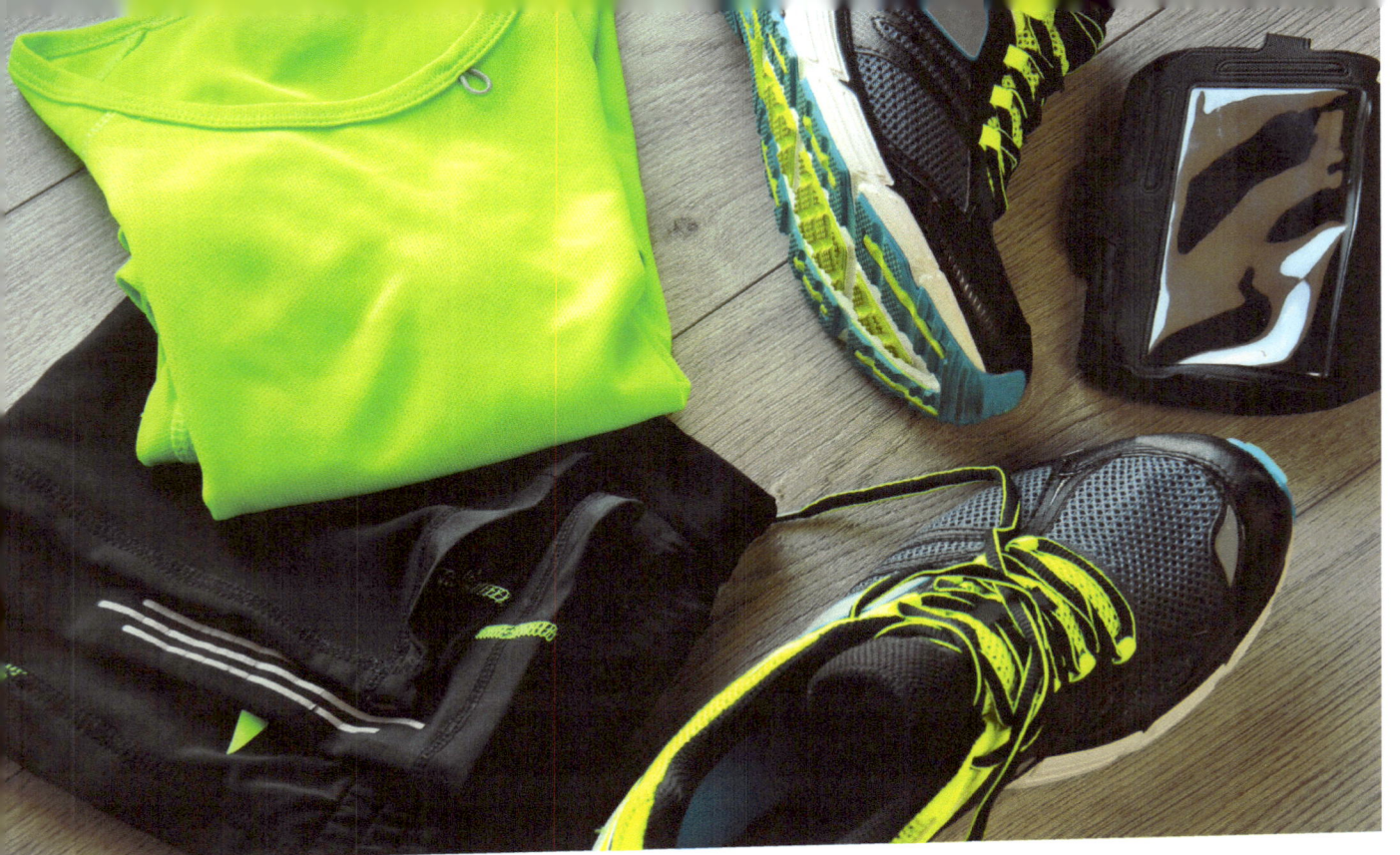

proper clothes to wear

One of the best things about exercise is that you can work out in simple clothes that feel good. Here's what to look for.

Wear shoes that go with the sport. Don't buy shoes that feel uncomfortable in any way. They should feel so good that you want to go out and dance! It is very important to get **professional** advice on shoes.

In **warm weather**, wear clothes that fit loosely and breathe.
These let air flow freely over the body, and more heat can escape.
In the summer, wear light colors. These reflect heat.

If your clothes get wet, don't change them. Wet clothes help keep the body cool as water evaporates during exercise.

In **cold weather**, wear clothes that cover not only the arms and legs but also the hands, feet and head.

Wear layers of clothes but not heavy clothes. As you warm up, a layer can be taken off before you sweat too much. As you cool down, you can add something back.

Change wet clothes in cold weather to keep the body warm.

Exercise and other health concerns

blood vessel disease (arms & legs)

This is known as peripheral artery disease (PAD). If you have this disease, exercise can be painful, especially in the legs. This does not mean that you can't exercise. Aerobic exercises using the arms and legs can help you build your strength and be able to do more. You can walk, cycle, row, do arm curls or other exercises. You can safely exercise until the pain is moderate to severe and then rest. After resting, start again. This is called **interval training.** Make sure your HCP knows which exercises you want to do. He or she can help you decide how much and which kind is right for you.

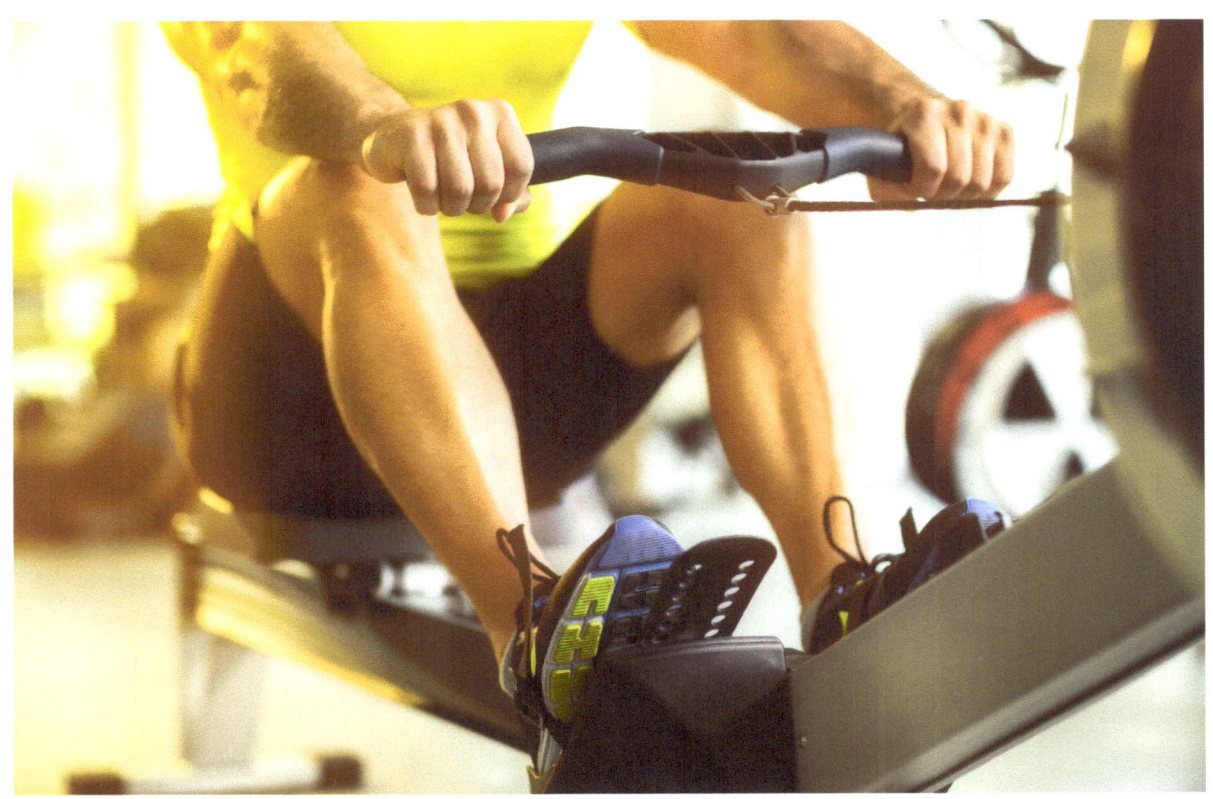

lung disease

Studies show that exercise can help people with lung disease.
It can build:

- **endurance** and **strength**

- **confidence**

As the chest muscles get stronger through exercise, shortness of breath may also improve. You can exercise even if you use oxygen.

If you know you have lung problems (scarring, fibrosis or emphysema), it is best to have an exercise test to see how much you can do.

diabetes

People with diabetes can exercise. It is now almost always prescribed as part of treatment. If you are diabetic, ask your HCP exactly which exercises you can do and how much.

You should not exercise when ill or when blood sugar is way out of control. This is most important if you inject insulin. You could go into *insulin shock* if you exercise at the wrong time. Always take some form of fast-acting sugar with you when exercising. Any exercising diabetic can be caught off guard by a sudden drop in blood sugar.

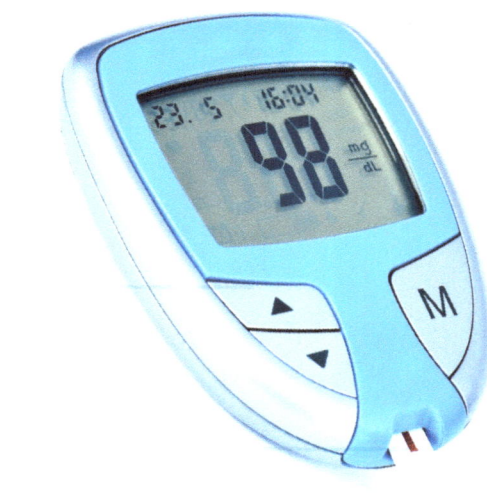

meter

blood sample

test strip

Exercise cautions

There will always be times when you should stop exercising. These are called **end points.** An end point may be muscle strain or irregular heartbeats. It can also be unusual shortness of breath or chest discomfort. No matter what it is, an end point tells you that it's time to stop exercising. If you train past an end point, your health could be in danger. An example would be someone who exercises even though he or she is having chest discomfort. The more you exercise, the better you know your end points and when your body is saying, "STOP!"

Sudden death, heart attacks and heat-related illnesses have been caused by vigorous, physical activity. But these are rare. These are almost always due to heart disease in people who:

- **smoke**

- have **uncontrolled high blood pressure**

- have **very high cholesterol** and **narrowed arteries**

- have a **family history** of early heart disease

- **exercise without knowing what is safe**

If you don't know how healthy you are, or if you know that you are prone to heart disease, have an exercise test. This is most important for people 40 or older who are just starting to exercise or who want to exercise more.

Do not exercise if you have chest discomfort, palpitations or an illness with fever. These should be evaluated by your HCP.

When you know you are at risk for heart disease, work out in a medically supervised program. In these programs, you have experts to help you lose weight, quit smoking and change your diet. They can also show you how much exercise is right for you. As you improve your health, you will be able to exercise on your own.

food, alcohol & drugs

Do not eat large meals or drink alcohol before exercising. Exercising too soon (less than 2 hours) or too much after eating puts a strain on the heart.

Alcohol, marijuana and cocaine increase heart rate and may affect the heart's pumping ability. They may also hide any symptoms or end points that are telling you it's time to stop. Over-the-counter decongestants can also raise heart rate and blood pressure during exercise. If taking these, you may need to decrease your exercise level.

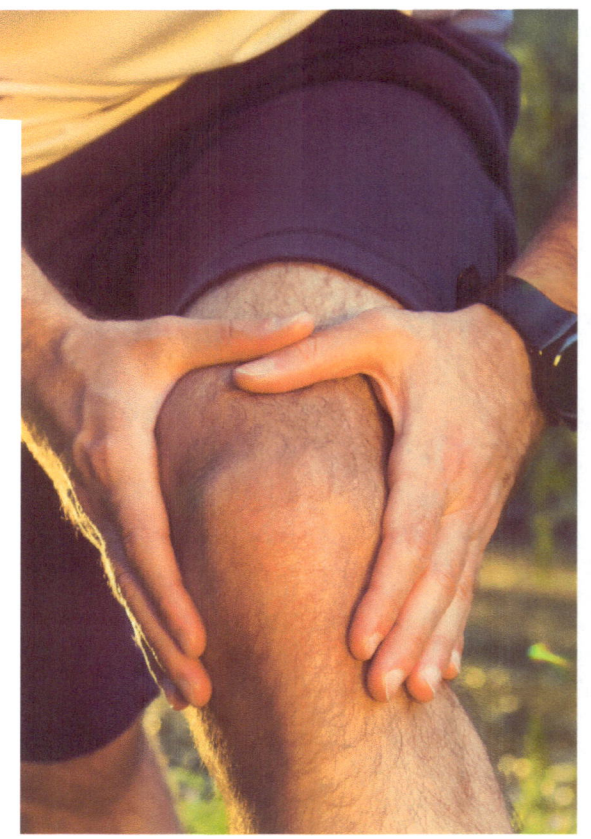

bones & joints

There is no evidence that lifelong exercise causes arthritis. In fact, it may make the bones and joints even stronger. Bone and joint problems are more common in people who:

- **do too much** exercise after a long time of no exercise

- have had joint problems before

- do not do stretching and flexibility exercises

- do exercise that is too strenuous

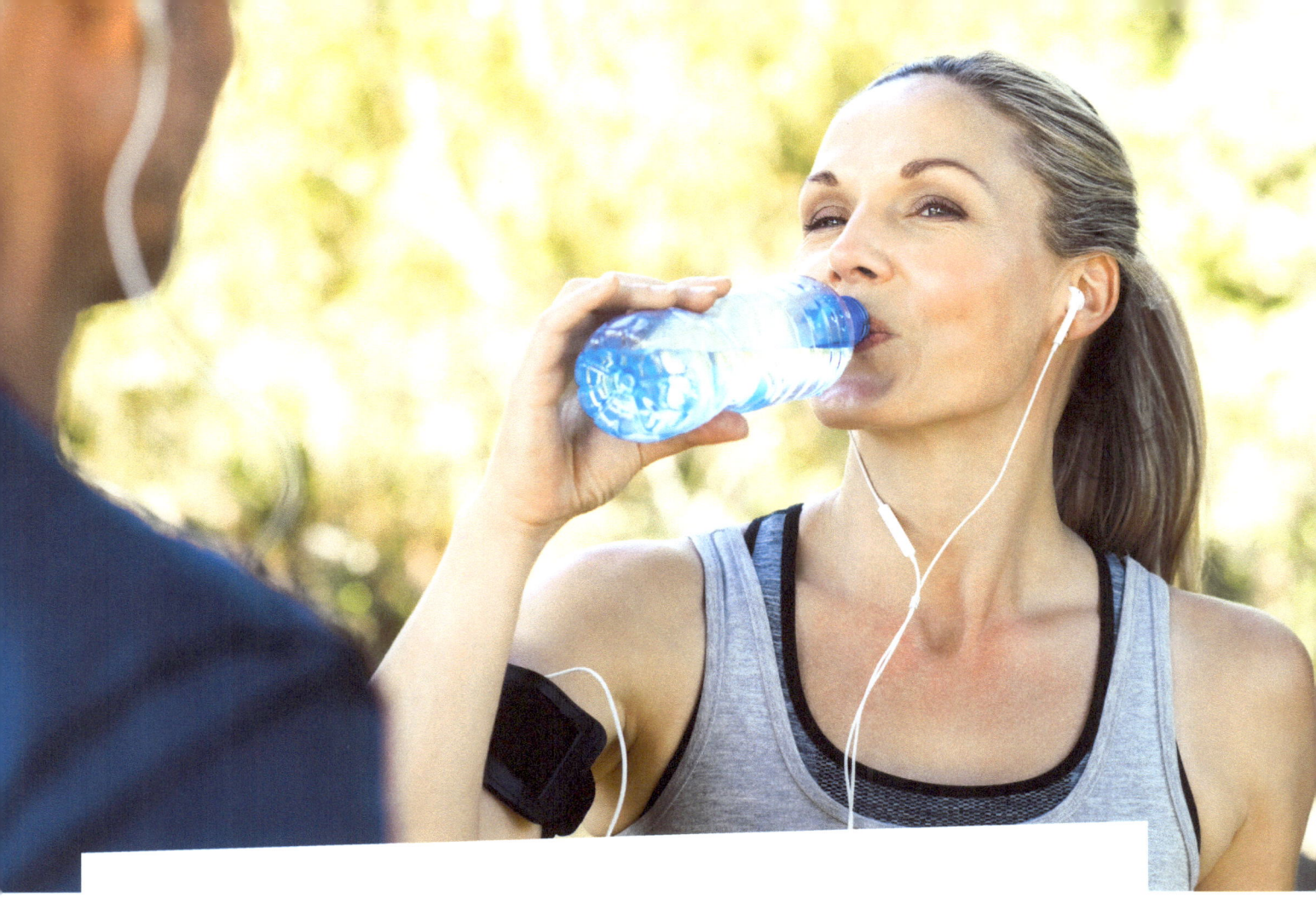

heat sickness

Heat sickness can happen with exercise. It can happen to:

- long distance runners not in their best condition

- people who are overweight, not trained or not used to heat

- people who do not replace fluids during exercise

- very young or very old people with previous heat problems

- people who increase their speed during the last part of an exercise session

These problems can be prevented with proper training and replacing fluids.

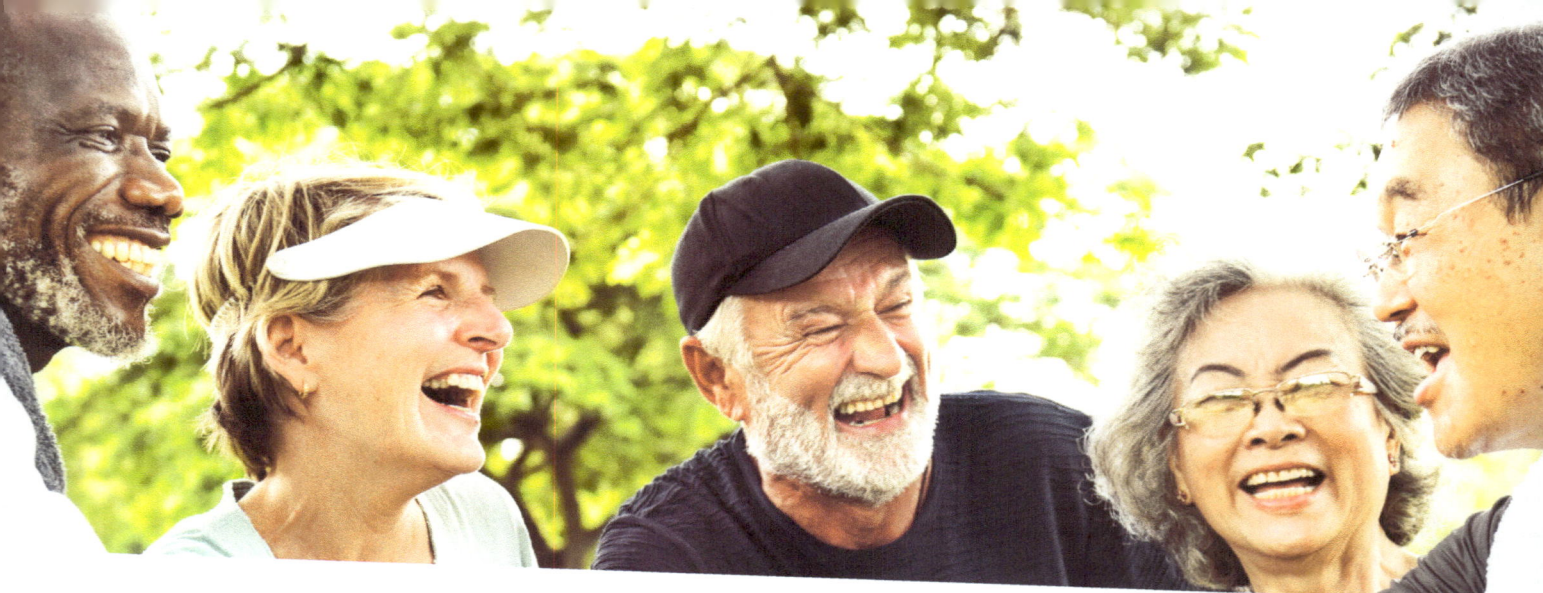

Summary

As you work to stay in shape, keep your health and safety in mind and remember these:

- It is best to get your healthcare provider's advice to begin or increase an exercise program.

- Know your target heart rate range and when to stop an exercise (end points).

- Warm up and cool down each time you exercise.

- Start with 20 to 30 minutes of aerobic exercise a day and increase to 30 to 60 minutes as you train. Do this most days of the week (5-6 days).

- Include stretching and flexibility exercises in your workout. These should be done after your aerobic exercise (3-4 times each week).

- Ask your HCP if you need an exercise test. This is important if you are older, have not been exercising regularly or have heart, lung or other health problems.

- Pay attention to heat, cold, humidity, altitude, surfaces and pollution.

- Do exercises that you enjoy and that you can continue the rest of your life.

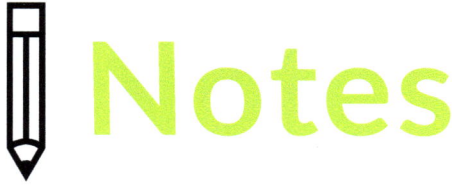# Notes

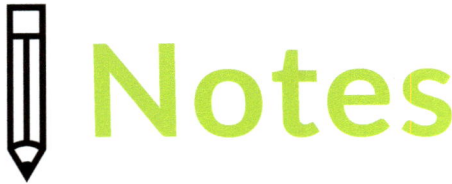# Notes

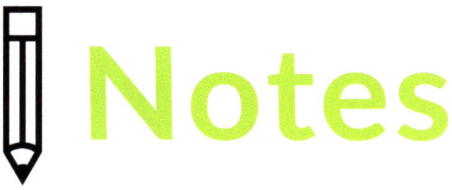

Notes

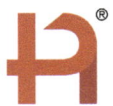